THIS IS NOT A SELF-HELP BOOK

Mark Mehigan is a comedian, writer and podcaster currently based in Dublin, Ireland. Whether selling out live shows or entertaining his many followers on Instagram with his weekly roasts, he is usually found having a laugh at the state of the nation today. After spending his early twenties working in the music industry as a songwriter and moving around a lot, Mark eventually 'settled down' and spent the remainder of his twenties going back and forth between London and Dublin, working in the BBC and hosting his popular podcast, *The Sunday Roast*. In 2020, Mark returned to Ireland full time where he bought an apartment in Dún Laoghaire before making the galactic leap to Castleknock where he lives now with his fiancée Doireann Garrihy.

MARK MEHIGHAN

THIS IS NOT A SELF-HELP BOOK

BUT IT MIGHT JUST HELP YOU

Gill Books

Gill Books
Hume Avenue
Park West
Dublin 12
www.gillbooks.ie

Gill Books is an imprint of M.H. Gill and Co.

© Mark Mehigan 2024

978 0717199945

Designed by Typo•glphix
Edited by Jane Rogers
Proofread by Anna Paterson
Printed and bound in Great Britain by Clays Ltd, Elcograf S.p.A.

This book is typeset in Elena Basic.

The paper used in this book comes from the wood pulp of sustainably managed forests. For every tree felled, at least one tree is planted, thereby renewing natural resources.

A CIP catalogue record for this book is
available from the British Library.

5 4 3 2 1

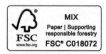

For Doireann, my family, my friends
and friends of Bill.

CONTENTS

INTRODUCTION

My name is Mark and I am an alcoholic. You could probably also call me a drug addict. Cocaine, specifically. And, of course, cigarettes. Most recently, Häagen-Dazs salted caramel ice cream and Haribo Supermix. The spectrum of things that I will sink my teeth into is vast. I'm addicted to anything that will separate me from myself, even if only for a moment. If it offers a brief holiday from my head and the never-ending ways my brain seems to work against me I'm likely going to be a fan.

As a child I was told I had an 'addictive personality'. I won't say that I'm addicted to everything, because that's not true. I'm not addicted to exercise. I've never been addicted to getting up early or doing the washing-up. I don't become preoccupied with the desire to be rigorously honest and I am not exactly hooked on expressing how I truly feel, especially if it makes me uncomfortable and might affect other people's perception of me. I have yet to become obsessed with apologising quickly or accepting constructive criticism from those I love the most.

I am mostly a fan of substances and pursuits that require little work but very quickly and very suddenly transport me into another place or feeling. Anywhere beyond the tedious quagmire that is the here and now. I'm always looking for a different dimension to *me*. I was not born with a desire to drink alcohol, but I do believe that I was born lonely. Sometimes it can feel like I was born four or five pints behind the rest of my friends. I'm just one of many people who came into this world without the gene, the organ or the bone that enables one to just *get on* with life. It was as if there was a missing part within me and I knew it from a very early age. Others had it. I lacked it. I didn't even know what 'it' was but I knew that I didn't have it. I felt different. I felt *off*.

Now, I don't mean to despair too early. I was

still a very outgoing child. I shouted a lot, I pulled faces, I made jokes. I got angry all the time. I was very precocious. A red-faced little extrovert. When people say a child is extroverted, generally they mean annoying, though, don't they? That's what they're trying to tell you. It's almost like a warning. 'Oh, you're going over to the Maguires' house? Their little one Cliodhna will be there. She's such an extrovert.' Translation: 'Enjoy the barbecue, mate, you'll be kept on your toes by that charmless little rat scurrying around your feet for the entire day.'

It's sort of like the person who says they just 'tell it like it is'. Have you ever encountered one of these individuals? They are the worst culprits of them all. What I find interesting is that they never seem to be *telling it how it is* about positive things. It's never about the good aspects of people's lives. It's never a comment about how happy you look lately or how much weight you've lost. No, it's always the negative stuff. And they say it with such pride. As if they're doing the universe a profound service by courageously *telling you it how it is* while the rest of us, apparently so shackled by the chains of convention, pathetically choose to keep quiet about odd haircuts, confusing fashion choices or ugly spouses and babies.

Nevertheless, I'm going to try to tell you *how it is*. But first, I'd like to make it clear what the purpose of this book is. It's not an autobiography. No, it's not one of those books that you usually see written by comedians with a title along the lines of *Joke's On Me, Now Who's Laughing?* or something else so despairingly obvious that it makes you wish they ghosted their ghostwriter after the very first Zoom call to discuss the project. I'm not remotely famous enough for one of those.

This is a memoir about drinking and an exploration of the relationship that I have with myself. A *then* and *now*, if you will, spanning most of the critical periods of my life. I hope this book will cover why my drinking began, how it got so bad and what it's like now to live without it.

When I first explored the idea of writing something serious, I had lofty, arrogant notions about penning *the* manual about modern alcoholism, deconstructing the taboo surrounding the word itself while also highlighting how invisible this disease can be – it doesn't always manifest in end-stage experiences of lost faculties, lost jobs or lost families. In my case, the thing I squandered most was my potential. And my wellbeing. And my job, actually. And a few relationships. And lots of money. And opportunities. And friends.

I thus set my sights on mapping out an instruction booklet for those who occupy the same space as me. There had to be others! Individuals who weren't near destitution, but couldn't stop fucking up their lives either. Those who lived in the undiagnosed middle ground of problematic drinking, the expansive grey area where partying might be a constant source of pain, with alcohol comfortably positioning itself at the centre of all of their woes, but somehow things never quite getting bad enough to stop completely, especially after comparing themselves to *real* alcoholics. I thought that if I wrote down where I went wrong, other young people might avoid descending into substance abuse and might even steer clear of the spiritual abyss that I found myself wallowing in for the many dark years of my twenties. I convinced myself that this was going to be the book about drinking. A righteous manual for life, perching itself nicely on the philosophical crossroads between *The Power of Now* and *12 Rules for Life*. Maybe I would become a vulnerable and more progressive version of one of those internet misogynists? I quickly got lost in a fantasy – which, as you'll soon see, is a tendency I have – in which my terminal sense of uniqueness knew no bounds.

But soon I came to realise that I am absolutely no authority on addiction. I'm not even educated enough to advise on it. I knew a guy once, a writer, and in his bio on Twitter he had written, 'A writer with a background in psychiatry'. His background in psychiatry was that he had been admitted to a mental institution three years previously after a bout of mania. Not exactly the same as a PhD from Trinity, is it? I think I'd sooner pay someone €100 to listen to my woes if they at least had an undergraduate degree, Brian. So I hesitate to claim to discuss addiction knowledgeably or to speak as if I am coming from a place of understanding on how this whole thing works. Just because I overdid it until I had to stop drinking, it doesn't make me an expert on willpower or a specialist in recovery. It's only been a couple of years since I was regularly poleaxed on bathroom floors, regurgitating the stomach contents of the day before. All I can do is talk about my experiences so far and how things went for me, both with my drinking and then in my recovery.

The earnest truth is that I would like to offer a little bit of hope. Or at the very least, present the argument that no behavioural pattern is truly unbreakable, no matter how long ago it was formed, and that it's not too late to change everything you thought you knew about yourself. I'm sure that some of you reading this right now might lack a sense of optimism for the future. Perhaps you are sick and tired of feeling sick and tired. When reflecting on the state of your emotions and the coping mechanisms you use to soothe them, maybe there is a concerning 'Why?' lurking just beneath the surface that you haven't addressed yet. Maybe the perceived bleakness of the world has become so familiar and constant that you've forgotten what it might be like not to be secretly miserable. That's what happened to me, anyway. It's quite easily done, really. Self-loathing and the old *hole in the soul* of addiction form quite a lethal combination. For too many years I lived without any optimism for the future and grew to accept that as normal. I felt like a prisoner in my own life, trapped in my own head. Stuck making the same mistakes over and over again, without any rhyme or reason. It was as if the outcome was predetermined. The game was already sewn up. I thought that I was simply designed to be a failure and destined to be a fuck-up. I used to drink to make myself feel less different from other people but in the end it was my drinking that made me different from other people.

Normal people don't go to a different corner shop every day just to ensure the guy who works there doesn't get the daft notion you've got a drinking problem.

The cynic inside me baulks at the idea of sharing my journey. It feels far too earnest, too self-indulgent. My mind tells me I am a fraud, an imposter. I have never climbed a mountain, I have yet to win a race. I wasn't born into abject poverty. Neither, on the flip side, have I ever attended university. I never got the English literature degree I thought I would. I never won a Grammy. I have yet to overcome any real form of external adversity or arrive at any destination. My life is still buffering. My life is incomplete. Pending, if you will. If my recovery from alcoholism is a peak for me to climb, I'm not even at base camp. And I will rue the day that I think I am. This book is not a guide to living and certainly not offering a solution to a drinking problem. I do not have any answers. Instead, I will strive to ask some solid questions. My only currency is my experience.

So please consider it less of a 'how to' book and more of a 'please don't'.

It's not all doom and gloom, but it *is* important for me to be honest about the lows I experienced and to discuss the places my drinking and drug use brought me, because the day that I forget that is the day I am fucked. I will do my best to ignore the imposter syndrome that has been molesting every part of my consciousness since I came up with the idea of the book and give it to you in a very honest way. The funny thing about my addiction is it wants me to start believing the worst things imaginable about myself because the moment I do that, it stands a chance. The moment I start to give air to all of the negative self-talk that tells me I am a piece of shit and totally worthless, it starts to win. Because once I start believing those thoughts, what's the point in anything? And if there's no point in anything, why not take a drink? All roads lead to Rome. No matter what emotion I am experiencing – good, bad or indifferent – I have to be careful. It's important that I stay alert to my own thinking and monitor my insanity on a round-the-clock basis.

This means looking at the myths that I had previously maintained about my character and the type of guy I was – self myths that I firmly believed to be true. Like this one, for example.

MYTH:

I enjoy the buzz of going to a big sporting occasion and look forward to the craic and atmosphere of the crowd.

REALITY:

I would prefer to go to the pub alone and get absolutely mangled while watching the Helsinki Under-9s compete in a javelin-throwing contest than head to the Aviva and watch an Irish match sober.

Learning about my *actual* personality has been one of the unexpected perks of recovery. And I'm still learning and unlearning every day. This is a book about addiction and it is a book about connection. It is my story and I hope you take something from it.

Oh, and before I continue I just wanted to clarify – this is definitely not a self-help book.

It really isn't. The title was not designed to deceive. Speaking of self-help books, actually, I've always believed you should only be allowed to write one. As soon as there's a part two or an 'updated' version, you've revealed yourself to be a complete spoofer, haven't you? I thought your first book had all the answers? I thought it contained the cure? I thought that pocket-sized spiritual 'cookbook' – with a curse word in the title – contained the magical recipe we need to live the perfect life?

You know the type of books I'm talking about. The non-fiction slop you'd buy last minute in a WH Smith because you've got a short-haul flight from Gatwick and it comes with a free Dairy Milk or bottle of Smartwater. The only reason you're in there in the first place is because you've got low battery and need to save some juice on your phone so you can order a taxi on the other side. So you go into the airport shop – which smirks at the concept of a cost-of-living crisis – and after negotiating the self-help aisle with an American wearing a confused expression and a literal duvet cover, you sift through the latest tat professing to offer enlightenment. Even though the 18-minute Ted Talk you crisis-watched on the Megabus didn't dissolve a lifetime of anxiety, perhaps one of these paperbacks will?

I was in the airport recently and there was a handwritten sign above a stack of books that said 'Contemplative Reads'. Have you seen the books they have on sale in these shops? *50 Ways to make a Polar Bear Sneeze, The Real Wolves of Wall Street* ... If we're calling the books in Dublin airport 'contemplative', we may as well award the orphanage Oliver Twist grew up in with a Michelin star.

Nevertheless, I generally opt for a book with lots of colour and a BIG BOLD TITLE with a colloquial tone, which I find totally irresistible. And then finally, after having my senses mauled for about 45 minutes on the plane, I put it down. And there it stays. Nestled between a chewing gum-stained sick bag and the laminated card explaining via cartoon how to busy yourself before you die if the plane goes down. And I return to my mind. The dodgy neighbourhood that is the residence of my thoughts. A place I was recently advised never to go through alone.

I was huddled under a doorway, having a cigarette with a couple of other alcoholics, venting about some micro-drama in my life and this man said to me, in a serene 20-years-of-sobriety-and-has-definitely-seen-it-all way, 'Mark, you're the type of person who responds to getting a flat tyre by slashing the other three', and I've never felt more seen in my life. He then went on to say, 'Your brain is like a bad neighbourhood, don't go in there alone. Especially at night. Pick up the phone and call someone before you do too much thinking by yourself.'

I used to scour the pages of self-help books with a feverish sense of urgency. Like a Hollywood detective in a classic whodunnit, tearing through a phonebook to see if the name he is searching for correlates with the address he has written on the back of his hand. Always searching for the answers. I never seemed to find them. They all say the same thing, these self-help books. Focus on what's within. Surround yourself with good people. Try to be more forgiving of yourself. Allow yourself to experience pain. You deserve joy and happiness. Get out of your own way and embrace the imperfections. Switch the phone off every now and then. Reconnect with nature. Remember it's okay to feel overwhelmed by life. By technology. By love. By everything. Suffering isn't endless. You are not alone.

Not what I wanted to hear, I'm afraid. I'd sooner drink dishwater from my grandmother's verruca socks than heed advice that tells me to sleep regularly, exercise often and talk to a professional. Give me something faster, baby. Don't make me work for it. I mean, I know they're right. Clichés become clichés for a reason. But when you're hurtling towards a nervous breakdown at the age of 26 and using payday loans to fund a burgeoning cocaine habit, you'd really like them to contain a lot less 'Be honest and discuss your feelings with friends' and a lot more 'Here's a sure-fire way to get rich financially, spiritually and mentally ... and all in time for the weekend.'

I used to love self-help books.

I would start them so optimistically. Like the first day of the school year. Fresh-faced and naive. Ready to change the world. I was always under the illusion in school that new stationery would transform me into a model student. It was all about the pens. A multi-pack of biros and a few new pads of A4 paper were exactly what I needed in lieu of knuckling down. My appetite to improve myself was insatiable and I was now armed with the appropriate tools to get the job done. I would be unstoppable.

Within a week I'd come home from school with one shoe on and a hole in my trousers so big that I may as well have been wearing crotchless tights. The pencil case would be long gone and I'd have resorted to signing my name with a jagged rock I'd found in the back garden. And that would be the end of it. It could be something as trivial as a burst yoghurt in the bottom of my schoolbag, and I would be throwing in the towel. 'Ah fuck it, I'll try again next year. All those teachers are assholes anyway.'

Of course I was going to love self-help books. Any form of quick fix that looked neat and required little effort. If I had grown up in America with access to infomercials I would have been completely fucked. There's a solid chance I would have overdosed on diet pills before my first communion or drowned inside a water bed on the night I lost my virginity.

I just don't understand self-help books these days. *How to Give Less of a Fuck and Get Shit Done.* Why are you cursing at me? Am I supposed to be motivated because you're using bad language? Do you think it will create an inspirational stirring in the gut? Oh wow. I've just been shouted at in capital letters. What a feeling! I'd better fix up immediately. Shoulders back. Neck straight. This book means business. It demands to be taken seriously. It's cursing. It probably drives a motorcycle. Maybe it hangs out in dive bars, shooting frames of pool with charming, venerable sex workers. It wears sleeveless gloves and refers to its wife as its 'old lady'. It has a bandana with an eagle on the front. It knows when to draw the line under a joke and not drag it out ...

'Give less fucks'? Oh, believe me, I've tried. I would love nothing more than to be freed from the chains of fucks that I have been giving since day one about what other people think about me.

I've never understood the concept of not taking life too seriously. I would have thought, surely, take it very seriously? Take it extremely seriously. It's literally the only type of existence you will ever know while inhabiting your current form, so I'd say take it very seriously. Unless, of course, you're one of those people who gets really into Ayahuasca and starts thinking that life is just an imagined concept for us 'sheeple' and you will have no role to play in it. Yet, confusingly, these people still seem happy enough to use their mum's debit card when they need to go to the dentist? Riddle me that, please?

I grew to loathe these self-help books and the sexy, empty wellness they espoused.

I found them inauthentic, almost white-labelled tokens of spirituality, filled with copied and pasted bastardised niceties cherry-picked from other more profound bodies of text. Their lack of depth would make your horoscope feel like the Mariana Trench. Astoundingly average suggestions on how to improve your quality of life and 'take back control'. I was looking for the opposite of that.

The most spiritually liberating element of my journey so far and the closest I will ever come to experiencing peace of mind is the moments when I truly forfeit control and accept that I have no control over anything or anyone in my life. That's where the money is, for me. Letting go and relinquishing that perceived sense of order. And not in a nihilistic sense. But with people, places and things. On the days I'm present enough to have the awareness that I have utterly no control over anything other than my own behaviour and how I choose to respond to the world, that's when I am the most happy. That's when I feel pure. That's when I am free. Life on life's terms.

An alcoholic said to me recently, 'I'm not to

blame for my first thought, but I am responsible for my second thought.' I found that an incredibly valuable tool to apply to daily life, both internally and also when it came to relationships. Allowing myself to experience whatever the first thought is, without blame. Let go of the guilt for whatever imperfect notion or idea has crossed my mind. But don't sit in it for too long. Don't stew. Accept it. Now I'm responsible for what to do with that thought. As somebody who suffers enormously from spiralled thinking and can very easily have one uncomfortable thought trigger an entire day of unwanted and tormented introspection, I really found that helpful. Whenever the 'this is how things should be' thoughts start creeping in, that's when I know I'm headed for trouble. 'Should' is a very dangerous word, after all.

I haven't figured out how to let go and practise acceptance all the time, either. But I have learned some things. And by the time I reached 30, it was certainly time to try anything at all that might lift me up out of the mire I found myself in. I needed a new way of living. I was broken enough to ask for help, and desperate enough to take it when it was offered to me.

These days I often hear people say, 'You need

to get out of your own way.' Whether it's offered reassuringly by a fellow former drunk or shouted down the camera lens on Instagram by a self-proclaimed entrepreneur who is undoubtedly both unemployed and also extremely uninspiring, I hear it everywhere. But there is some truth to it. A large part of my recovery entails identifying and then deconstructing the various myths that I maintained about myself and the world around me. Until I stopped drinking, I never realised that I had such a rigid outlook on life, such a skewed perception of the way things were. It turns out that I was wrong about pretty much everything! Life on the other side of the walls I had spent years constructing to hide behind is more colourful and beautiful than I ever could have known. Reaching out and asking a stranger for help when I needed to stop drinking was the catalyst for everything changing, and marked the first moment of my existence when I realised that most of the self myths I held were totally untrue. I quickly learned that help is available.

Generally, people do want to see you do well. Usually, fewer people have written you off than you think to be the case. Most of them aren't even thinking about you in the first place. There are others like you, and to be truly alone is a decision rather than a reality. For too long, I defiantly assumed that life would always be the same, with my happiness trending downwards and the chaos trending upwards. The very first time I spoke to another alcoholic, he asked me if I was actually ready to stop drinking for good. I said yes. He then told me something which I have yet to find a circumstance in life where it doesn't apply: If nothing changes, nothing changes. If I hadn't acted during that moment of desperation in 2021, when the tsunami of drinking and despair was about to sweep me away for good, everything would have remained the same. I would have continued on that trajectory, slowly isolating myself from the ones I loved while at the same time believing that it's all that I was worth and all that I was good for – as if drinking and snorting my way into an early grave was what I deserved. In the end, by asking for help I was finally doing something different and unknowingly changing the course of my life for ever. These days when I am arguing with somebody or myself, I try to remember, 'If nothing changes, nothing changes.' There is absolutely no point in engaging with the world in the same way I used to and expecting different results. It won't happen. True change requires a genuine transformation of attitude and the daily application of new behaviours. It's not easy but for me it's all about breaking the chain. Only then can the magic happen.

You know the way in movies, when someone gets shot they often don't realise how badly they've been hit until the gunfight is over? They're in the getaway car and all of a sudden the cherry-red stain appears on their white T-shirt, and the life begins to leave their eyes? That was like my twenties. I just had to keep going because I knew if I stopped for long enough to assess the damage, I'd probably never get up. I just had to keep going and keep dusting myself off after every minor scuffle with reality, or close call with my rock bottom, until finally the ground went from beneath me. And I gave up. I couldn't do it any more. I just couldn't.

I started to see the value in some of these self-help books.

So if you're worried about your drinking, read on. If you're interested in hearing about my drinking, read on. If you're in an airport and wondering why you didn't buy *F*&k the B*lls**t, Be Your Own Boss, Bi*ch*, I've got nothing for you,

I'm afraid. At the end of the day, I'm just another middle-of-the-road drunkard who gave it a good old lick until the internal dereliction became too much to bear. I was sick and tired of being sick and tired. Ultimately, I would just like you to know that everything *genuinely* can get better. Life as you know it can transform within an instant. There is an existence beyond your comprehension sitting patiently at the end of a request for help. Although, it has to be said, circumstances can also get an awful lot worse too. Even rock bottom has a trap door and the crazy train only stops when you decide to throw yourself off it. So please make your mind up and start the process of sorting your shit out, will you? Nobody else is going to do it for you. Unless the burning inferno of a car crash that is your life ends up spilling over into other people's lanes and disrupts their flow of traffic, you're probably going to be left to your own devices. The intervention I was waiting for never came.

CHAPTER 1

UNCOMFORTABLY YOUNG

Some alcoholics I know talk about the intense feeling of bliss that comes with their first sip of beer. That was not my experience. My descent into problem drinking was slow and painful.

Like a story from your mother about how she got from the airport to the hotel when she went on holiday. One of those ones that goes on for so long you can't quite remember where it began and you don't know if it's ever going to end. All you know is, at some point, you sort of 'come to' and realise that this is your new reality.

My alcoholism took many people by surprise. And they weren't the only ones. I was blindsided too. How the fuck did this happen? I wasn't even one of the *bad* ones growing up. I didn't start drinking until I was 14. Most of my friends began at 12. The astonishing cliché of people assuming that in order to be an alcoholic one must be horizontal on a park bench, sipping from a brown paper bag with a skull and crossbones on the front rings true. In fact, since I got sober, I've even had a few people tell me that I am *not* an alcoholic. I think some people would like to be presented with a certificate of insanity from the local asylum before accepting someone may have an issue with the booze. Until they see me getting chased down the dual carriageway by two men holding butterfly nets, I simply need to 'rein it in'.

But look, that's none of my business. I don't want to focus on them – and let's be clear, this book is not an attempt to *prove* to anyone that I am an alcoholic – but I think it's interesting that many of us have preconceived notions of what it takes to be one. I was the same. I thought that until I drank in the morning, I didn't have a problem. Until I crashed a car, until I lost a job, until the girlfriend left me, until I slept beneath an ATM or crouched beside the toilet in the cubicle of a train station, draining a miniature bottle of vodka just to endure the morning commute, I was not a 'real' drunk.

The never-ending, miserable catalogue of 'not-yets' that I desperately clung on to as justification to continue drinking.

My poor relationship with alcohol likely stemmed from the poor relationship I had with myself.

Like many works of Irish literature, it began in a field. Well, almost. It began on a riverbank. It began before I was ready. I hadn't started drinking yet but my friends all had. It wasn't nice. I remember feeling like this whole thing was happening far too soon. It was reminiscent of the afternoons spent with the older cousins in my granny's back garden when I was a child. There'd be a game happening and I would desperately want to be involved. But before I'd even had a chance to ask how to play, everybody would be running to their hiding places and the captain would be counting down from 30. 'Wait, please, can everybody just slow down? This is all happening far too fast and I don't know how to play yet.'

I was slow to understand the concept of drinking. Only two weeks beforehand, we were watching wrestling, wearing cartoon-themed pyjamas and having sleepovers. We still had bedtimes. Yet suddenly I was expected to know the difference between a naggin and a shoulder, which cigarettes tasted the best with cider and where to put your fingers if you found a willing partner on the dancefloor. It sounds funny but it was fucking terrifying. I hated it. This loud onslaught of adulthood. With its dick measuring (often literally) and fist fights. I felt betrayed by the friends I thought I had. Since when did they care about these things? Why didn't they tell me or give me fair warning? The metaphorical water rose and suddenly I was struggling to stay afloat, just to keep up. How did everybody know about this stuff? It was as if everyone else had been given the instructions. The blueprint. The manuscript. They all knew *how to be*. American television in the nineties had lead me to believe that puberty lasted a few years. In Ireland I think it lasted five minutes. It's like we all went to sleep one night as children and then woke up at the age of 14, collectively dying for a cigarette.

Not for the first time, I found myself buying into the self-conceived and destructive idea that everybody else had their shit together and I was the only one who hadn't. It's a feeling that stems from self-obsession, I think – the inability to look beyond myself and see things from the perspective of others – because of course the reality was very different.

MYTH:

Everybody else knows exactly what to say and how to act. They get it.

REALITY:

Nobody knew what they were doing at 14. I know some of the guys I was in school with might claim otherwise, but absolutely none of us were experts at fingering. In fact, it's probably something that most of us still struggle with, even in our thirties. Everybody was carrying a healthy amount of teenage fear and busy mimicking behaviours they had learned from their older siblings or cousins in order to fit in. I wasn't the only one with a sense of outsiderness.

This myth that I was the one *not getting it* and that I was the one on the outside would plant the seed of fear and self-doubt in my brain that I would then spend the next few years carefully watering.

So – the first night I ever went to a 'drinking' disco. Early in the evening, we went down to the banks of the River Dodder. Which sounds an awful lot nicer and much less heroiny than it really was. You'd be forgiven for thinking it sounds pleasant. I mean, when you say 'banks of the River Seine', it evokes the image of sophisticated Parisians wearing berets and sipping cheap but delicious wine, gesticulating while discussing philosophy or politics. The activities on the banks of the River Dodder were a lot less poetic. One time I was given a joint to smoke that was filled with my friends' pubes just so they would have a story to bring back to the other guys in our class on Monday.

Another time I saw a guy trying to defecate into the top of the Lucozade bottle. And it was a squeezy top.

The part of the River Dodder that we frequented was like most city centre shorelines. Decorated with abandoned shopping trolleys, used syringes and discarded condoms – the holy trinity of urban decline. A solemn place mostly visited by heroin addicts, teenage drinkers and closeted homosexuals. I remember walking through the bushes and the undergrowth, worrying what would happen if I got a nettle sting, because usually Mum took care of those with dock leaves. I was still a child. The others seemed so cool. So calm. It was as if they had been doing this all their lives. I was on the fringes. Looking over their shoulder as they marched into the decrepit opening between the bushes. I was tense and apprehensive. What happens now? I didn't experience the euphoric rush of rule-breaking or any sort of giddiness in my stomach. I just wanted to go home. I didn't, of course. The risk of not falling into step with the lads and furthering the feelings of isolation far outweighed any of the internal angst or instinctive urge to flee. I needed to be a part of it, whatever it was.

I was surprised by the mundanity of the drinking itself. Much like with a fist fight, all the excitement seemed to lie in the build-up. The planning. The anticipation. The filthy, primal excitement of what might take place set a standard of expectations that reality could never meet. Once the actual guzzling got under way, it was all fairly uninteresting. I watched the boys drink cans of Druids cider and discuss which of our teachers was most likely to enjoy adventurous sex – or at least whatever version of sex our 14-year-old virgin minds deemed adventurous. Probably just sex, to be honest. And then they got drunk. And they started chanting. Sports songs, pop songs or whatever other guttural sounds they could produce in unison that vaguely resembled a melody. I tried to get involved but I just couldn't bring myself to do it. I couldn't shake off enough 'self' in order to let go and join the so-called choir, while standing on the river bank with the muddy water making its way through my shoes until my socks got wet. I was far too aware of myself. Far too aware of my body. How I might look. Far too aware of my voice. How I might sound. I used to loathe it when groups started chanting. The aggressive birdsong of teenage boys. Angry and afraid and bulletproof and clannish. I could only contort my personality so much. Much of this is still the case.

You see, even when abiding by all the 'rules' and mimicking my way into social circles, I often ended up on the outside. I felt like I was always falling short. I now know, of course, just how wrong I was. Every teenager deals with these feelings at some point or another. I am not unique. But at the time, I thought it was a monumental character flaw and particular to me. I'm embarrassed to say this, but I used to literally pray at night that I would wake up in the body of my older brother or another one of the boys in class.

Anybody but me. It's hard to intellectualise these feelings at the age of 14 to the extent that you might be able to tell someone about them. At that age, it's just a feeling. Like joy or irritability or hope ... this *outsiderness*. It's just something that you 'know' and it slowly becomes part of you. Being different. Feeling *off*. Not knowing why. Yearning to be with the rest even though you don't identify with them. It's desperate, really. I wasn't comfortable in my skin from day one.

If I knew then the ease and comfort that I would one day receive from drink and drugs, I would have started a lot sooner.

* * *

I started getting panic attacks when I was 15. I still remember my first one. It was grotesque and sudden. It felt like I was getting shot in the chest with a cannonball. Jelly legs and unspeakable, breathless despair. I thought I was going insane. One minute I was fine and then the next

I wasn't. I really, really wasn't. I was sitting in the back of science class. I looked to the person sitting beside me, David, and said, 'I am going to die. Please call an ambulance.'

In that instant, the consciousness that I had experienced up until the age of 15 was annihilated, and the version of life that I had had pre-panic attack was gone. It was over. Imagine switching from colour TV to smoke signals. The force of the fear that swallowed me up that day was like an electric shock to the brain that sent my mind into convulsions. It sucked the breath from my lungs and the life from my face. I was buckled. I was fucked. I didn't know what was wrong but everything was wrong. Something terrible was going to happen and I was at the heart of it. I was being pulled down beneath the waves and I was going to drown. I remember watching the documentary *Blackfish* on Netflix about five years ago and seeing that harrowing scene in which the killer whale toys with the trainer in the pool. If you haven't watched it, one of the torture techniques the whale deploys throughout the ordeal is holding on to the trainer's foot and pulling him down into the darkness below. The trainer can't breathe. But every now and then, the whale drags him back up to the surface. For almost long enough to draw a breath. But then he's gone again. Back down to the shadows. That's what it felt like. To this day, I think my first ever panic attack was the most terrifying experience of my life. (Until the next one I get, of course.)

I'm genuinely even sweating here today, 18 years on, as I think back to it. The strangest thing about panic attacks is that there is an eerie familiarity to the physical sensations that wash over your body. It's a 'known' feeling but for all the wrong reasons. Like the warmth that spreads across your sheets after wetting the bed. Or when the sides of your mouth fill up with saliva before you vomit. An unwelcome familiarity.

You'd think that after a few panic attacks you'd get used to the sensations and learn to expect (and accept) what happens. But oh no. For me, anxiety has a funny way of materialising in a new and improved way each time. So every time I have a panic attack, my brain says, 'Oh wow, well this is very different from all the other ones before. This is *sure* to be the one that kills you.'

I suspect it's similar to those who have experienced the grief of losing a loved one or, to take a more mundane example, the searing agony of extreme dental pain. Only those who have suffered a full-blown panic attack will understand its weird and unpredictable horrors. Sometimes I wonder do I even have panic disorder or do I just suffer from PTSD from experiencing that very first panic attack? Who knows.

Now, I want to stress that I am not assigning full blame to the fact that I have anxiety. Yes, it was certainly on the list of ingredients that formed the recipe for my alcohol misuse, but it would be disingenuous and categorically incorrect to pluck the metaphorical strings of the violin and say that I only drank due to anxiety. I drank for a thousand reasons and I drank for none. Was I anxious because I drank or did I drink because I was anxious? They're not mutually exclusive. Ultimately, there is a much deeper, spiritual reason for my addiction that is so complex I will probably never be able to wrap my head around it, so we won't lose sleep over that for the moment.

My fear, anxieties and 'outsiderness' as a teenager manifested in a myriad of ways. I mean, of course there was a general spiritual malaise, a feeling of being ill at ease with myself and the never-ending, unwanted introspection. But there were also practical, daily inconveniences that anxiety brought about. Things like extreme bouts of hypochondria, panic attacks, doctors' visits, insomnia, chats with counsellors. Fear permeated every facet of my life. In hindsight, I can say it definitely contributed to me being difficult. I was a tricky person to be around at times. Considerably more supercilious than even the rugbyest of the rugby lads in my year, I looked to emulate the behaviours of those who were socially successful, but I never seemed to pull it off. I was the opposite of a wallflower. Gregarious, outrageous and hot-headed. A ludicrous enough individual and an expert at concealing my vulnerabilities.

I started regularly engaging in therapy when I was in my late teens. It helped almost instantly when it came to understanding my panic attacks and anxiety, so I quickly started using the sessions as an opportunity to perform and entertain instead of getting better. Oftentimes I would just list off the various people who I felt had slighted me in the previous two weeks. There were many. Back then, I thought that 'having a shrink' was an emblem of deep intellect and would often skip down the path to my appointments – they offered a 60-minute window of completely uninterrupted self-exploration. It's funny now, when I reflect on some of the things I used to say to my therapist. It was never going to work. I treated the whole situation as if I was the troubled protagonist in a coming of age movie. I didn't take it seriously. I would regale stories from the schoolyard or pass comments on someone else's personal life for 55 minutes before briefly revealing the cracks in my own thinking, spitting out something desperately vulnerable before marching out and chain-smoking three cigarettes in a row. Some days I would almost expect my therapist to ruffle my hair playfully at the end of a session and say, 'Go on, get out of here, ya little scamp. Oh, and hey – try not to break too many hearts this week!', like some sort of female version of Robin Williams in *Good Will Hunting*. Therapy is good and in my eyes should be mandatory for everyone, but for many years I just didn't take it – or myself – seriously enough to approach it with the right mentality. I was unteachable. Several years later, I would learn that until I got really honest, no amount of counselling sessions would help me. Rigorous honesty is the only tool required to conduct a thorough excavation of self, and without that, there's just no point. For much of my life I thought that because I could express myself well when it came to discussing other people's emotions I never needed to take a deep look at my own.

My academic tenure could best be described as 'colourful'. School was something I endured rather than enjoyed. My mother still says her greatest achievement to date is getting me through the Leaving Cert year. Some children who feel out of sync with their peers like to keep their heads down and just get on with it. They burrow themselves in the library and quietly form friendships away from the mainstream, discovering who they are while ignoring the loud, belching zeitgeist. I did the opposite. My way of dealing with feelings of inadequacy were to chase popularity and seek validation from students and teachers alike. But if I didn't get the results I desired, I would quickly lose interest and become very destructive.

I was told recently that hurt people often tend to hurt people and it makes a lot of sense to me. At times in school I was the victim, and at times I was the perpetrator. My popularity fluctuated, and so did my weight. I will always remember after one particular falling-out with two friends, there was a period of time when I couldn't sit at a single desk in the entire school without seeing the words 'Mark is fat' scratched into the surface. It scratched me a lot deeper than the surface. My response was to lash out at those I deemed weaker than me. It felt powerful to use some of the anger I had at myself for being the way I was and to take it out on other people. One time a guy merely tackled me the wrong way in PE, and I stood up and punched him straight in the face. Totally unacceptable. Kids are cruel. I was one of them.

It's complex and confusing how little empathy we can exercise when fuelled by fear.

Looking back and remembering my obsession with Eminem as a younger boy, I can now very easily understand how the likes of Andrew Tate and other internet misogynists manage to culti- vate large followings. I would have been a prime target. I didn't like my teachers. I didn't fit their mould of what a good student was and they would regularly remind me of that. I couldn't seem to find a consistent rhythm with my classmates. I wasn't happy at home either. I was disruptive but felt misunderstood. I frequently lashed out at others, which likely made me a very difficult person to sympathise with and thus furthered my initial feelings of isolation. When I see the state of the internet today and the culture of extremists – in all their iterations – preying on naive young men who are susceptible to influence, I feel very lucky that back then the internet was just illegal music downloads and the occasional pair of tits. It was a simpler time.

Somewhat speaking to the above, anger is much more attractive than fear. This is still something I need to constantly work on. Although anger may be my first reaction to a situation, there is usually a much more vulnerable emotion lurking beneath the surface. Sort of like a break-up in your early twenties, isn't it? The allure of masking the pain with anger. It's a lot easier to head down to the pub and say, 'My ex-girlfriend is a complete psycho' and dish out a few manipulated anecdotes to prove it than confront the fact that you are just a bit sad, and don't quite know how things got so bad so quickly, and stayed that way for so long.

My parents got separated in the summer of sixth class, which affected me enormously. Between that and the aforementioned self-loathing and increased social uncertainty, I developed a derisive persona that would take more than one book on drinking to dismantle. Anger was easier than fear. You probably noticed the reference to my weight. It would be remiss for me to write a book about identity issues and the disconnect that existed between me and myself without discussing the relationship I had with my body.

It feels strange and uncomfortable to talk about body issues, so you'll have to bear with me. Maybe it's because of my gender. Maybe because I am not *extreme* enough. I do not have an eating disorder and I never did. In fact, my way of dealing with weight-related self-hate was to eat more. I would gorge on shite when I felt shite. I still do. So I would rather not offend those who do live with disordered eating or vaguely allude to understanding the suffering they endure. It's interesting, though, that even now, as I write this, it amazes me how my mind can totally comprehend the spectrum of addiction when it comes to discussing alcoholism, but for some reason is incapable of applying the same logic to food 'stuff' and body issues. I feel like an imposter, a fraud. As if I need to be *qualified* to mention my own experience. Madness. It makes me wonder how many people aren't getting the help they need for fear that they exist too much in the grey area and do not merit the attention of professionals. Or that they may get laughed out of a doctor's office should they find the courage to open up about their concerns? (You won't get laughed out of anywhere – book the appointment!)

In any event, when I was around 10 or 11 years of age, I started putting on weight. Some people called it puppy fat. Some people called it fat fat. It happened almost overnight. I went from being a 'wee slip of a thing' to one of the three 'fat' guys in class. It became the first insult I heard in the schoolyard and the last thing I thought of at night. I still have a vivid recollection of crying in the bathroom mirror when I was about 12 years of age, squeezing myself in the stomach and saying 'You stupid fat f**k, why did *you* do this to *me*?'. I wasn't only angry at being fat. I was angry at *myself* for letting myself get fat. And there is a difference. It's only now that I wade through the waters of recovery do I realise that.

Every time I was stung by the radical honesty of the schoolyard, I would make a quiet promise to myself to stop being this way. I would become skinny, immediately. Surely it's possible to lose a few stone by tonight? *Be less like me and more like others.* Alas, September rolled around with its school bags and uniforms, and I will never forget the shame of being measured, only to discover I had a bigger waist size than my older brother. The lazy lack of awareness shown by the seamstress in the school section of Arnotts, who remarked loudly that although I was only 12 years of age, I had the waist size of a 15-year-old. It absolutely crushed me.

Throughout these years, I fervently ignored my studies and became a bedroom fantasist.

From day one I wanted to be a musician. It was quite simple. Or so it seemed. It was all I ever wanted to do, really. Somebody recently said to me that his entire basis of spirituality and willingness to believe in a power greater than himself ultimately stems from the human ability to feel the beauty of a sunset or to experience the power of music. We don't know why we find ourselves in awe of its beauty, we just do. There isn't any science that offers a reason, but we don't need one in the first place. Logic isn't required to know how we feel. Certain things just move us. I discovered rap music when I was about six years old (Eminem, of course) and it was like discovering the answer to a question I hadn't even asked yet. Rap had everything. I was obsessed with the words, turns of phrase and rebellious wit. Growing up, I enjoyed being funny, sarcastic and being quick with a come-back. Rap music had all of that. Rhythm, bravado, fantasy, escapism, the want for more from life than what you already knew – the leafy suburbs of South Dublin, lol – and an inherent sense of struggle that, for whatever reason, resonated with me. With that, the Spice Girls posters were ditched and thus began my lifelong relationship with music. Throughout my teenage years, I'd spend the evenings writing essays, songs and angry poetry in my bedroom. Dreaming of being in a different place. I also played the guitar and dreamed of becoming the next Eddie Van Halen in order to travel the world. Take me anywhere but here. I didn't realise what was happening at the time. I didn't know that the itch I perma-nently felt was not one of the geographical kind – no amount of 'anywhere' would scratch it. *I would always run out of road.* I think it's important for me to use the word 'fantasy' here, by the way, because 'fantasy' would ultimately play a huge role in my drinking. The whole notion that this time things might be different kept me drinking for a lot longer than I should have done. The idea that one day, somehow, I will be able to drink like a normal person. There *will* come a time and I will be on the Riviera with an Aperol spritz, skinny and happy, with my hair slicked back, and able to go for two drinks before retiring for the night. This is a total illusion and it must be shattered by taking stock of every single ugly reality I faced in the years when I drank. No amount of abstinence will result in a physiological, psychological or spiritual shift large enough to enable me to process booze normally. I am an alcoholic now and for ever. The invisible line was crossed at some stage. *C'est ça. C'est tout. C'est fini.* The option to drink is no longer on the table. To try and go at it again is to reject my entire way of being. It is to say no to life and yes to pain.

It wasn't always like that, though. I drank 'normally' for most of my teenage years. In the sense that I got black-out drunk most weekends, in the middle of the afternoon, and took to the bed by 11. Drinking just like the rest of my peers, in public parks and playing fields. Random beaches and abandoned houses. It didn't seem like an issue at the start. Usually somebody would overdo it and have to get their stomach pumped. Others would go missing. Someone got hit by a car once. There would always be a bit of crying. It's utterly bananas, in hindsight, when I think about how normal it was to drink the way we did. And how often we did. I don't want to express any sort of 'Sure, look, it was no wonder I became an alcoholic'-type sentiment, because that is not how I feel, and neither is it the truth. The vast majority of my peers who engaged in the exact same drinking back then are absolutely fine now when it comes to booze – but, Jesus, it makes you wonder.

I struggled with finding my 'place' socially throughout my teens. The classic 'too much of a jock for the nerds and too much of a nerd for the jocks' predicament. Or, more probably, 'too nice for the assholes and too much of an asshole for the nice guys', depending on which way you look at it. Bizarrely, the fear of having to get my stomach pumped or getting arrested by the Garda Síochána would always have been dwarfed by my fear of being rejected by 'the group'. A word I still hate. The elusive 'everybody'. It got bigger once we reached third or fourth year. A mixture of schools and sexes. This large, heaving mass of drunken teenagers moving through the suburbs. The only time it was ever referred to as a group was in the context of saying who *wasn't* in 'the group'. Once you're in, you don't talk about it. You're just in. And that's fine. But when you're not in the group, you're *really* not in the group. I craved that feeling of belonging. Being part of the crowd. The more I chased it, however, the further I went from achieving it.

When I was 16, I went through a growth spurt which would help shed the excess weight I had been carrying. That was not to be the end of those issues, though. Very recently, actually, I found myself back in a therapist's office, working through the difficulties I have been having with my body after quitting smoking and putting on a bit of weight.

The old thoughts have come creeping back to haunt me. 'You're a fat piece of shit and won't be of any worth until you lose the weight. You're an embarrassment.' *Be less like me, and more like others.* It's a setback I wasn't expecting, but again, anxiety and my addiction work in mysterious ways. And that's okay. I've learned that now. It's okay for it to ebb and flow. But we can get to the philosophical stuff later.

When I was 18 years old I moved to Brighton to go to music school. It was then that I discovered daily, habitual British drinking. I was lonelier than I would ever admit to myself and started buying cans of Foster's from the corner shop in the evenings to keep me company. And for a while, it worked. It really, genuinely worked. The pub was my passport to escaping myself and for a long time it did its job. I found my crowd. But the lifeboat would soon become the storm.

CHAPTER 2

FAKE IT TILL YOU BREAK IT

By the time I got to the UK, I was already exhausted. I was only 18 years of age but surviving secondary school had me feeling like I'd lived through a war. I probably should have taken some time after school to breathe, to dust myself off and to process my next steps, but that was not my style. I wanted to be out in the world *right now* and away from Dublin immediately. Bizarrely, I managed to sit a half-decent Leaving Cert – a D3 in ordinary level maths and an A1 in higher level English – but it was of no consequence. I wanted more from life, something bigger, and studying English literature and media studies in D.I.T. was definitely not the answer. I was convinced that a fresh country with new people – something exotic – would be the perfect solution to all my problems. I had always been a fiend for the shiny and new. My experiences of growing up in South Dublin had convinced me that the issues I encountered over the years were due to the personalities I was forced to be around rather than anything going on inside. I was of the teenage and hideously clichéd opinion that everybody in my school, family and area were simply too closed-minded and clannish. If I wanted to be happy, I would need to surround myself with cultured souls – open-minded artists and free-spirited musicians. Surely then I would thrive? Ironically, I resented the very upbringing that had afforded me the luxury of choice in the first place. In all my wisdom, I just wanted to run.

I spent a few weeks working on my parents until they relented and agreed to support me in moving to Brighton to study music in a 'new' college. It wasn't exactly a university, but it would get me a diploma in songwriting. Now, aside from the fact that a diploma in songwriting is probably as valuable as a wheelbarrow of Greek drachmas in late 2009, we must remember the important part – it was something different and it would get me out of Ireland. And so I set off to conquer the world.

Reality hit me in the face like the heel of a Doc Marten. Within three weeks of arriving in Brighton I was out of my mind with homesickness. Anxiety gnaws, hangovers bite, but loneliness swallows. It's a heavy sort of sadness that turns everything grey and blurs life into one large, monotonous blob. It starts in your feet first thing in the morning. Like water filling up the boots of a sailor in the hull of a sinking boat. Then it stays with you throughout the day, until finally presenting in its fully formed, ugly madness at night. To this day I don't know why I found it so difficult to pick up the phone. It felt like it would be a defeat of colossal proportions. To admit that maybe I was wrong. To accept that I was a bit lost. To confess that I seemed to struggle to do all the simple things that my peers could, and, ultimately, that maybe moving here was a mistake. Before I moved to Brighton, I felt as if I had spent my whole life staring out of windows; in the classroom, on the bus, in the back of my parents' car, yearning for the day I could eventually call myself an adult and actually exist in the 'real' world. Yet here I was and I hated it. Everything was happening too fast again. The weekends were the worst. They stretched out in front of me with their empty infinity and I had no idea what to do with myself. Sometimes I would buy the newspapers that my parents read back home, in an effort just to feel more connected to them. And partly because I genuinely thought that's just what 'adults' did at the weekend. A copy of the *Racing Post* and the Weekend section of *The Times*, tiny fragments of home, left unread on the table in front of me, as I sat in a café, staring out of the window.

Brighton was a strange enough place through the lens of my 18-year-old self; before then, my idea of hedonism was a glass of red wine and a cigarette while having a pretentious conversation about Wes Anderson movies outside a Parisian café; whereas the incense- and hemp-smelling damp bedsits of Brighton was the reality I faced. The drugs of choice were weed and meow meow (mephedrone). I didn't partake in either. I lived across the road from a Wetherspoons and every Saturday night there would be fights with the 'DFLs' – Down from Londoners – spilling onto the street after a day of watching the footie. Hooligans, essentially. One time I saw a guy using the hubcap of a car wheel as a weapon, like a real-life version of Oddjob from James Bond. Odd*yob*, perhaps? It was the first time in my life I became aware of my privilege and just how protected I had been from that 'real world' that I spent my teenage years yearning to be a part of. From an artistic perspective, Brighton was a sort of spoofers' purgatory, with an eclectic tapestry of musicians, poets and general 'crusties' forming the fabric of the coastal town. I quickly realised I wasn't quite as bohemian as I once thought. Which is the story of my life, really – existing in the grey area. I was writing music and running gigs around town but I still didn't feel part of anything. I struggled to connect. Again, I found myself on the outside. Mostly through my own doing, of course. The opportunity to create friendships was there but, bar one or two, I kept everybody at arm's length. I wanted so much to be part of a gang, but my understanding of how social circles worked had been massively distorted by my experiences in secondary school. Note to reader: applying the social dynamics of a private school common room in South Dublin to anywhere else in the world is going to be a disaster. For example, greeting someone you've only met once with

'What's up, baby? Heard you've got a small dick!' probably won't come across as charming as you think it will. Especially when the girl has taken a 40-minute bus ride from Eastbourne for the sake of this second date.

In my first year there, I was living with eight strangers in a dilapidated five-storey house that had rats in the kitchen and holes in the floorboards. One night, a lovely Greek Cypriot housemate, who we'll call L, suffered a severe episode of psychosis followed by a complete breakdown, which resulted in him fighting the police in his bedroom, before being subdued, sedated and carried out of the house in a makeshift wheelchair. He had been battling his own demons, and had spent the previous few months closed off in his room, isolated and smoking weed. It seemed the weed had eventually turned on him. He had drawn bullseye targets all over his body in permanent marker and I remember catching his vacant stare as he was carried out. It was quite traumatising and I was totally out of my depth when it came to managing the situation. I tried to enlist the help of guidance counsellors from our school, but they were non-responsive. I remember trying to explain to his parents back in their home country, via his aunty, who could speak English, that their son had been sectioned by the police and was currently being held in a mental health facility up in Chichester. I had never even heard the term 'sectioned' before that night. I got the train up to Chichester the next day to see him, with one of my other housemates, James. His room was under guarded watch. The whole thing was terrifying. James hugged me in the car park and we both started crying. Then we went drinking. I only ever saw L once after that, when he came down with his aunt several months later to collect his belongings. And then he was gone. I wasn't the only one struggling.

Aside from that, there were also minor, youthful misdoings that would create the occasional issue for me to try and fix. Just before the Christmas break in first year, I made the exceptionally asshole mistake of sleeping with the older sister of another of my housemates. She was visiting for the night, after taking him on a trip to IKEA. I spouted just enough believable bullshit for her to think that I was more mature than I really was and I played just the right amount of Bon Iver songs to appeal to her 'studying-English-literature-in-London-and-in-search-of-a-great-big-romance' stage of life. And we got together. She swore me to secrecy about our late-night rendezvous, and of course I gave her my word. I felt bad when I told everybody in the morning, but I could never let a promise get in the way of a good story. And that sort of encapsulates exactly who I was at the time. I wanted to be *better* but I couldn't resist the temptation to receive validation, regardless of the moral compromises needed to get it. It became exhausting, waking up in the morning and making a solemn promise to myself to behave a certain way, only to find myself slipping back into toxic and comfortable habits by lunchtime. I hated it, but I couldn't seem to help myself.

It was around then that I started drinking alone. Less than some, more than most. The corner shop was my dispensary. Eight cans of Foster's and a one-pound frozen pizza. Almost every night. A solemn liquid supper for the burgeoning problem drinker. It quickly became routine. The vast expanse of a Tuesday evening could either be spent negotiating with ennui or filled with a quick 'fuck it' and a night of swallowing beer. It almost felt poetic. I lashed out at my loneliness by pouring alcohol on top of it, in an attempt to drown it. *Maybe if I just ignored it, it would go away?*

MYTH:

I couldn't have a drinking problem as an 18-year-old – going on the lash is what students are supposed to do. If I just acted like it wasn't a problem hard enough, maybe it wouldn't be?

REALITY:

It was here in Brighton that I cemented the destructive belief that you could outrun, outthink and outwit your own problems. This would never, ever work, no matter how many times I tried it in the future. Like a wasp at a picnic or an aggressive panhandler, this was and still can be my instinctive reaction when facing a challenge – exercise forthright indifference to the fact that it's even occurring and soon it might dissolve. I wouldn't recommend it, to be honest.

In any event, even though I had started drinking a couple of years before, it was only in Brighton that it really began to take. This time it was different. It was medicinal and it was with intent. I was drinking to *counter* a feeling rather than to create one. Previously, I had consumed booze as a mood enhancer, surrounded by friends and mostly just to fit in. Alcohol had been the gasoline to throw on an already raging fire of teenage exuberance, hormones and sexual anticipation. Now, however, I was drinking in an attempt to put the fire out. This one burned differently. I was anxious, irritable and restless. This was steady, purposeful self-sedation.

I easily adjusted to the new drinking diet. It was so gradual that I barely even noticed it. There would always be someone up for it, you see. The pubs of Brighton boasted many genres of outsider and I drank with most of them. I avoided the student bars because I felt I was superior to them. More mature. More worldly. Such was my fallacious arrogance that I presumed their pleasure to be infantile. I wanted to be with the older people. The cooler people. The wiser people. Not these ones, the other ones, just around the corner. Not here, *there*! They might have the answers, you see? I was always searching for the next thing.

One particular subset of people I encountered on my escapades were ex-London bankers who had been sent out to pasture by the seaside. Self-styled 'post-breakdown' City boys who now hung their heads in Hove, wandering along the seafront in jaded, jittery comfort. The sea is therapeutic but I often wondered if they needed something more rigorous. One person I remember in particular was Giles, a man I befriended. He was in his early sixties. And he wasn't a pervert, by the way. Because I know that's what you're thinking. He was just extremely lonely. Much like myself. Giles was probably an alcoholic and I was quickly becoming one. We went around the various pubs of Brighton together and he would listen to me talk about how famous I was going to be, and that the music I would eventually make would change the world. In the end, I think I changed my number, and I never spoke to Giles again. This would be a common occurrence in my life. The transient and fleeting relationships in every place I lived. Short, evanescent and intense partnerships only to be abandoned like the cheap T-shirt that shrinks after one wash, so you bin it without a second thought.

My life brimmed with many different iterations of Giles. A friend in every port, a port with every friend. A smorgasbord of outsiders. Drunks. Musicians. Lunatics. Oddballs. The occasional goth. Unified by the one great, unspoken secret that we were only *really* keeping from ourselves. The pub became my sanctuary. It was my clinic. I quickly learned the language. And there is a language to the pub. It's universal and it transcends class, gender, race and creed. It doesn't really matter who you are or where you are coming from. The drinking part of the pub was a haven for those who wanted it. It was egalitarian to its core. Belching louts and businessmen. Criminals and day-trippers. Milkmen and barristers. I fucking loved it. Other drinkers reading this will know what I am talking about. You could be anywhere in the world, but within five minutes of being in a pub, you are home. Forgive the hideous cliché, but I cannot explain it any other way. The culture of a pub is something I still miss. It's a different type of connection. Shared with grunts, nods and small talk over cigarettes, it was the perfect antidote to life. In the pub, time stood still. And that is a feeling I had been chasing my entire life.

Alas, the persistent drinking had my panic attacks and anxiety at an all-time high and within a few months I presented at the NHS to tell the doctor that I thought I had a drinking problem. Even the bottomless horror of a panic attack can sometimes have positive repercussions – it was likely the thing that propelled me to make the call in the first place. Either way, I knew that drinking was the cause and was worried that I couldn't stop. I never phoned home or told my parents what I was going through, but maybe a doctor could give me a quick instruction booklet on how to drink normally so I could enjoy pints like the rest of my mates. At this stage, I had made a few attempts at abstinence but never got more than a couple of nights before reverting to the old routine. I sat down in the clinic on Western Road with clasped hands and prepared myself for the interrogation. The doctor first asked me how often and how much I was drinking. So I told him the honest truth. And as we all know, the 'honest truth' in this scenario is when you take the number of drinks that you actually drink per day, minus that by at least three, and then desperately try to remember the number of units that go into each pint of alcohol, and ultimately offer up a figure somewhere between all of that and the daily recommended intake that won't immediately get you locked away in a padded cell. He then nodded pensively: 'Well, Mark, I don't think you are necessarily an alcoholic yet, but your drinking is definitely problematic. Unless you make some drastic lifestyle changes I think you will likely get yourself into trouble soon. I am also quite concerned about these untreated panic attacks, fluctuating moods and general feelings of anxiety that you mention. I highly recommend you ...'

Yes! It was the greatest news I had ever been given. I was *not* an alcoholic. My passport to continue on this journey had been issued. He then droned on for a while about moderation, therapy and all of that nonsense, but my head was already gone. Thinking about the beers that night. Staring out of the window ...

The inclination to overly poeticise these formative drinking years is something I will try to avoid. At the root of it, of course, there were the reasons outlined above. But there was also another fundamental truth at play – I loved going out on the piss. Let's call a spade a spade. It wasn't all teary-eyed bedroom drinking and sobbing into pillows, not even remotely. In fact, lots of people reading this will remember me exclusively from the innumerable, outrageous binges and sprees. There were lots of good times. It took a long time for the drink to really turn on me. There were teenage summers spent at Puck Fair in Kerry, frequenting the pubs of Killorglin. There were French exchange trips in the banlieues of Paris and the beaches of Biarritz, ordering ten meals at Disneyland because you were only allowed one beer with a burger and chips. I was lucky enough to go to Los Angeles during the summer after sixth year and it was so good that I still experience euphoric recall when I think about watching The Chemical Brothers live at Electric Daisy Carnival in the University of Southern California bowl. That summer of 2009 before Brighton was essentially a joyous three-month bender that peaked with watching Moderat perform live at Electric Picnic in what was still one of the greatest live music experiences of my life. (Second to seeing Eminem at Punchestown when I was a chubby 12-year-old with bleached blond hair ... The only thing that's changed now is the blond hair.)

Before trouble came mischief, and there are countless examples of good fun that all came from drinking alcohol. I remember a time in fifth year in school, when myself and two other guys went up to the Montrose Hotel in Stillorgan, where we were supposed to be representing St Michael's College in some sort of national table quiz, only to leave due to the excess volume of nerds (in our opinion). We walked across the road into UCD, where we would end up drinking with 'college girls' in their dorm all night. Fun was had during my formative years and good memories were made. At the age of 18 you can get away with inhaling pints for 21 days on the trot without your bowels falling out of your ears and losing access to the wains. You can be bulletproof as well as breakable. There was a lot of indulgent mayhem. And it was great craic, too. The gap between what was happening inside my head versus the personality I put out into the world was only beginning to appear. I was cocky, bullish and oozing self-assurance on nights out. There was an arrogance that ran parallel to the suffering, too – I believed I would simply outgrow my problems. Maybe if I spoke loud enough, people wouldn't hear the tremble in my voice?

And so I ran with it. I leant into it all. I let myself become that character. You know the type. We've all encountered one. The guy who drinks and judges and dismisses his way through life, because it's a lot easier than trying. It's easy to be a character. You can get away with almost anything in your twenties too, I think. It's very easy to drink excessively while still untouched by the consequences of time. The unbecoming effects of constant boozing can fly under the radar as offshoots of youth – flakiness, constant drama, fluctuating moods – rather than clear signs that you might have a problem. At times I even convinced myself that my drinking was merely age-related and saw no reason to hold back. So on I went, hiding who I really was behind cigarettes and alcohol. Slowly letting the shutters come down on other aspects of my personality, leaving them in the dark, where they could not grow. This is the role I chose to play.

The cracks showed quickly in Brighton. For example, even with a generous allowance, I was still finding myself permanently broke. I just never had any money. It was gone before I ever knew about it. To this day I don't know if it's as a result of alcoholism or undiagnosed ADHD. Or maybe I'm just a sloppy kind of guy. I slept on a single mattress, without a bed, for nine months. Sometimes I would go to sleep hungry. I would spend every cent I had on drinking and when the money ran out I would borrow more from friends. And if I couldn't borrow more, I would try to get credit cards or sell my belongings.

Completely insane carry-on. For months I avoided visiting my aunty in Swindon because I couldn't afford the train fare. I remember one particular time going to one of those CeX electronic stores with my entire DVD collection, in a desperate attempt to get enough cash to keep me going for a weekend. A friend from Ireland was visiting and I didn't have a penny to my name. I must have had about £400 worth of DVDs in my rucksack. The cashier offered me about 19 quid for the lot. I was appalled. So I took it. Of course I did. Life was already becoming quite unmanageable and dysfunction was surfacing. And I still had a good 10 years of pain left in the tank! In hindsight, I wish I could shake myself and say 'Speak up, you idiot! Say something! It's okay to be afraid! You're 18! You don't need to know how the world works, nobody really knows how it works! Stop pretending you know what's going on!' But it was too late. I had committed to the bit. I thought I knew everything. I was also probably unable to even articulate how I was feeling. My problems felt too vague and existential, too internal. How do you pick up the phone to a loved one and just blurt out, 'Eh, basically, I fundamentally feel different from everybody else around me and I really wish I could rewind the clock back to when I was around 12 because I feel like this is all getting away from me quite fast and it feels like everything is out of hand and it's too late to change it ... Also could you please transfer me €100 for my flights at Christmas?'.

Although there was a lot of real-world chaos that began to pepper my time in Brighton, this is a diary of the internal rather than a catalogue of the external, and war stories won't bring me any closer to peace or understanding. Even the funny ones. In all honesty, it would be a while before it became properly noteworthy anyway. Such is the progressive and bewildering nature of this condition that it's not always fireworks from the start. I got a solid few years out of drinking before it got really bad. And there were some incredible memories made along the way. But there was definitely something in those early days in the UK, when my relationship with alcohol cemented itself as a permanent one and the booze became an extension of me, that it truly felt like a turning point. Going forward, it was going to be a case of fitting life into my drinking rather than fitting drinking into my life. That much was clear. A transformation had taken place and I wasn't yet in the business of correcting mistakes. I finally had something worth hiding. I was obsessed with drinking. All my life I had struggled to adjust in the way other kids my age seemed to be able to. It felt like I had to try extra hard just to be 'normal'. It didn't come naturally to me. The flow of life. But now, finally, I had something that made me want to embrace being different. I had a 'thing'. When I was drinking, I was glad I was weird. I had my flow. I had *arrived*. This period of my life would herald the beginning of the longest war I would ever wage with myself – the battle of wanting to be accepted, loved and to feel like I belonged versus the desire to be different, a thousand miles from convention and to exist anywhere else but here.

After just under two years in the UK I decided to call it quits on Brighton. (My version of calling it quits, as it happens, would be to come home and tell everybody how happy and successful I was.) I hadn't reached the dizzying heights of superstardom that I thought I would, and I suspect the people around me had grown a bit tired of my bullshit, too. Running gigs and open mic nights while presenting an internet-based music show called *Balcony TV Brighton* wasn't exactly the nomination for a Grammy or invitation to Los Angeles by a major label that I had dreamed of receiving in my first year in England. I did get offered a small record deal by an independent bedroom label that came with a £400 advance, but it was never going to work. I had fallen out of love with my life down there and I was sick of everything about the UK. I took the money for the record deal and never even signed the contract. I was ready to go back to Dublin. My incessant desire to be somewhere else at all times struck once more. I was done. It was Brighton's fault though, *not mine*. The world wasn't twisting itself into the shape that I desired and it was time to take this one-man circus elsewhere. On to my next location. This would be my second geographical. The aforementioned illogical belief that switching locations will solve all of one's problems, when in fact the problems are rooted in the person.

I'd like to say that I moved back to Dublin with my tail between my legs and a fresh sense of humility, but that is not the case. I was welcomed with open arms but I never opened my mouth. I arrived home with a bigger ego than I left with, a bitterness at my own perceived failures and now the makings of a drinking problem. Good stuff. At this point I think it would be remiss if I didn't say this: there are times when I reflect on my time in Brighton and I wonder 'Could things have been different if ...', but that type of thinking is not helpful to my recovery and it is ultimately incorrect. I knew what I was doing. Nobody grabbed my hands and wrapped my fingers around a pint glass. I had a family at home who would have moved mountains to help me if I needed it. Lord knows they did at other times in my life. But instead I chose to chase the elusive feeling that I found in alcohol. It was my desire to escape myself that brought me to the UK. And that desire would outlive the Lanes, the sticks of rock, the open mic nights, the Pete Doherty wannabes and every other musically doomed child of the Mumford & Sons era I came across in those days.

I barely said goodbye to the friends I had made in England. I thought my ability to just move on and change direction at the drop of a hat was a sign of strength. It was a sign of fear. In a predictable air of conceitedness, I felt it was more glamorous to up and leave, without so much as a farewell pint. 'They'll probably think

I'm going to greener pastures. Moving on to better things.' I had come to England to elevate my career, to achieve musical recognition and to live a much larger life than the one Ireland could ever have offered me. But in the end, I was flying back home, wounded and crestfallen, and the only thing I was leaving behind me in the UK was a Hansel and Gretel-esque trail of unmanageability. Notices to pay council tax, overdue phone bills and a rake of jaded friends – lots of the common trimmings of any modern alcoholic struggling to keep the plates in the air.

The more I reflect on my past, the more it makes perfect sense to me that I ended up an alcoholic. Of course it does. Richard Curtis couldn't conjure up a more romantic pairing. I was a restless teenage fantasist, and while living in the UK I discovered the one magical elixir that could help take me away from myself. It was always bound to happen. You cannot run for ever. You will eventually get tired. And when you do, you may need something to help you sit with yourself. That was the case for me, anyway. I spent my entire adolescence constructing a personality based on what I thought other people would like. A personality I thought they wanted. *Show them anything but you, Mark.* I was almost disabled when it came to being myself. My biggest fear – in the internal galaxy of millions – was that other people would see me for what I really was. A scared child who didn't quite know how to get along. So I ran from myself. I hid behind several layers of sarcasm, cynicism and emotional indifference. *If I don't care, they can't hurt me.* These character traits were the bricks I used to build a personality. And these bricks became the walls that would eventually imprison me.

And just like that I found myself back in Dublin, surrounded by my peers who had just finished university. Again I existed on the periphery. They beamed with insouciance and camaraderie. They planned holidays. They joined teams. They grew up. They *belonged*. I didn't match their tempo. So I did what any pleasure-seeking, young lunatic would do, and I got involved in the nightclub business.

CHAPTER 3

NEW YORK, SAME ME

Alcoholics are often experts at camouflage, and for many years I was no different. I never concealed my drinking; I disguised it. I hid my excess in plain sight. It was such a big part of who I was, so intertwined with my personality, wrapped up in my character, that it would have been impossible to separate the two. All my work, all my socialising and every one of my romantic pursuits came laden with booze. In fact, it was only when I met Doireann that I realised that around 90 per cent of my sexual experiences up until the age of 30 had occurred while I was under the influence. Now, I don't think I'll do any of my former love interests a second disservice by reminding them – and every other reader – about the details of those fleeting encounters. That's the least they deserve. Especially you, Sarah.

I arrived home from the UK at the age of 20, wounded and ready for a change. I would never admit it at the time, but the two years in England had starved me of the sarcastic, familiar and abrupt nature of Irish people, and I was actually quite happy to be back. The over-the-top familiarity of a local taxi driver asking you where your father worked or for the details of your mother's bra size was a welcome change from the deeply impersonal and formal nature of British life. I don't say that with any anti-English sentiment; I just found it staggering how vast the difference is in communication styles between Irish people and our nearest geographical neighbours. I always perceived a certain coldness to the inconsequential encounters of British shops and other mundane environments that I never adapted to. That wasn't the only aspect of my life in England that I was ready to shut the door on either. The previous 24 months had been far too introspective, too isolated and too inward. I felt I was too young to have a drinking problem and that by moving back to Dublin I was giving myself a chance to outrun the uncertainty I felt within. I wanted to outgrow those meddling feelings of unease. My way of doing this was to throw myself headfirst into the party scene at home. In a very deliberate and very Irish display of emotional suppression, I merely put the head down, ignored the bad thoughts and kept going. I remember thinking to myself after Brighton, 'Well, that was all a bit mental!' and simply moving on. I convinced myself that I only drank the way I did in Brighton *because* of Brighton. It was nothing to do with me.

I started going to pubs and gigs, knocking around other creative types who were interested in similar music to me. Just beyond the goths, All City Records was a record shop and label in Temple Bar owned by Olan O'Brien that was pretty much the epicentre of cool music stuff that was happening in Dublin. By day, it attracted an eclectic mix of heads – people also into hip hop, house music and beatsy stuff, along with graffiti artists, DJs, photographers and most other types of creative. I was never a regular pilgrim to the place, but I clung on to a cousin of mine long enough to get familiar with the lads in there and was introduced to lots of people 'on the scene' who then became good friends. We formed bonds over our shared taste in tunes and love of going out on the piss. I had a lot of fun. Most of my school friends were still going on college nights out and drinking cheap vodka around kitchen tables. They were busy growing up. But I decided to skip that stage of life, to press fast forward and move onto the next bit. It must have been an overcorrection to the fear that I used to hold about getting left behind. School had also instilled in me such an aversion to the mainstream that I never wanted to set foot near normality or convention again. I was ready to be an adult *now*. Going out to a student nightclub for €3 Wednesdays after sitting on a party bus and singing along to Flo Rida on the radio was my idea of hell. I would sooner have opted for a lobotomy. I wanted a *sophisticated* high. As it happens, it would quickly transpire that my interpretation of a sophisticated high would basically mean drinking in pubs instead of houses. That was the extent of it. But I convinced myself that what I was doing was worldly. I believed that maturing differently meant hanging around suburban beer gardens with my best friend, Stuart, chatting to problematic 40-year-olds about their love lives, or lack thereof. That's what separated me from the other kids my age and that's where I did my growing up. I thought I had it sussed. Most weeks would consist of jumping between various social groups – the school friends, the music friends, the town friends, the older friends, the new friends, until eventually on Sunday night I'd pick up the phone and call Stuart, trying to cajole him into coming out for a few *quiet* pints. We have been mates since we were 14 and our friendship is one of the few constants in my life that I am eternally grateful for.

It was in Dublin that drinking became my sport, my leisure and my personality. It gave a sense of meaning to the mundane. A two-hour chat in the smoking area of the Leopardstown Inn about *The Shawshank Redemption* and I'd be thinking, 'Yep, that was a solid enough Tuesday.' Acting 10 years older than I was, and 20 years older than I felt. I probably wasn't fooling anybody other than myself but it helped me to discover my role after school a little bit more and to figure out the makings of an identity. It doesn't come as easy for a young man when sport is out of the equation. Humour was a very protective shield, too. Regaling many 'well, here's a good one for you' stories to strangers, such as the time I met a middle-aged woman in the Lanes of Brighton, who wanted me to hide behind the rocks down by the beach and pretend to attack her, so that herself and her husband could wank to it afterwards. (This is true, by the way, although I only got as far as the seafront before getting too cold to continue. I was also fiercely afraid of what might be lurking down beneath the rocks at that hour. Not realising, of course, that it was *me* who was lurking down by the rocks at that hour.) I was a proud atheist and wore my lack of spirituality like a badge of honour. I mistook nihilism for depth, hoping the rest of the world would too. If you were to solidify the amount of shite I spoke in pubs between the years of 2012 and 2015, it would result in a fatberg three times the size of New York City. (If you're not already familiar, please do not google what a fatberg is.)

I had pub friends and I had club friends. A diverse collection of characters who helped scratch the various itches I needed tending to. If I wanted deep, meaningful conversations that occurred on barstools, I had friends for that. If I wanted the garish, loud, locker-room banter of a nightclub, I had friends for that, too. I moved between groups and gangs, hovering on the peripheries, adopting the desired persona to fit in, depending on the day. At the time, I put this down to me being a social animal. I was a man of the people. I thought it was merely a case of me being such an interesting guy that I required a number of different outlets for the diversity of my personality. Now, don't get me wrong. I *was* a people person. And I still can be. My appetite for meeting new and interesting individuals is one that I'll never sate. However, in this instance, the only glue holding my entire social network together was alcohol. And that would continue to be the case, across the board, for over a decade. None of my relationships was centred on a hobby or an activity that required anything other than getting out of your mind. I did not meet any of these people sober. I wouldn't have liked a lot of them if I did. And vice versa. When X friends would be having an off night and doing something mundane, like going to the cinema, I would go drinking with Y people on their night out. This compartmentalisation of my life would quickly become the modus operandi. All of my relationships, neatly tucked away in their own little boxes, each of them receiving a different part of me, depending on the day and what I was willing to give. From afar, I would just look like a gregarious party boy, talking shite everywhere he went. And, of course, that much was true. But I was also meticulously holding every single person I met at arm's length, for fear they might see the real me. The infinite balancing act, moving back and forth on a unicycle, trying to juggle the balls of life in the air. It became so exhausting.

It's very hard to figure out who you are when everything you do is an attempt to escape yourself.

I was trying to achieve success in the music industry. Parallel to my partying, you see, there were dreams, there were relationships, there were plans and there were ideas. I wanted to 'make it' in music and had dreams of doing comedy full time. It wasn't all black and white. I was still a somewhat functioning individual with the ability to do things, meet people and form bonds. There was an entire life unfolding at the same time as these drinking habits were being formed. The problems on the outside were only in their infancy. At a distance, it would often have looked like I was happy. At times, I absolutely was happy. There were bursts of success, flickers of change and moments of breakthrough. It's the non-linear nature of this whole thing that convinced me that I was okay, and to keep going down this path, ignoring all the warning signs. As far as I was concerned, my life did not resemble the life of an alcoholic, or at least the movie-like understanding I had of what an alcoholic is – a bearded vagabond shouting obscenities into his hands. I wasn't even close to that. I just enjoyed a few pints. I was a young creative, writing tunes and trying to make a name for myself in the music business. Drinking just came with the territory, didn't it? I was a *character*, you see. Somebody who enjoyed a laugh and a bloody good knees-up.

In order to earn a crust, I then got involved in the tawdry world of nightclubs. Because of course I did. Because where else would a 21-year-old with no college degree and a fiery passion for drinking go to make a living? It made perfect sense. Nightclubs were lurid, superficial playgrounds and the perfect hiding place for someone who wanted to drink every night of the week, no questions asked. The mainstream club scene in Dublin in 2012 left a lot to be desired and I was delighted to get the opportunity to disrupt the regime. I got a phone call from a guy called Anthony Remedy, who owned Andrews Lane Theatre at the time, and jumped at the chance to do something with him. He had heard about me through friends and thought that perhaps I'd be the right guy to spearhead a new Saturday night in the city centre. I created a brand called Brooklyn Zoo that threw hip hop parties and it quickly became quite successful. The name came from a song by the pleasantly named and venerable rap legend, Ol' Dirty Bastard of the Wu-Tang Clan. I took a tongue-in-cheek approach to the marketing of Brooklyn Zoo and spoke to the prospective punters in their own language, which turned out to be extremely effective. There were queues around the corner from the very first night. This was great for the ego and bad for the drinking, or bad for the ego and great for the drinking, depending on which way you want to look at it. I was earning a lot of money and I couldn't spend it quickly enough. My phone was off the hook with people wanting to be friends, to go drinking, to hang out. Next to going viral, there is no 'fame' more fleeting than being a nightclub promoter at the helm of the *in* spot in town. And I loved every minute of it. I was making crazy money for a 21-year-old, with no shortage of people to enjoy it with. I leapt into the available chaos that sudden access to money can bring. If you want an example of how quickly it all went to my head – one time I wore a white blazer on a night out without any irony. I was *that* demented. I drank every night of the week. I would stay in five-star hotels at the weekends. I would bring mates out for steak dinners on a Monday. On a couple of occasions, I would show up to the airport drunk and fly to the first place available, with the resident DJ of Brooklyn Zoo, Willo. It was a crazy, outrageous, hilarious and awful time. All at once. The speed at which I was living did not feel sustainable.

Some other concerning behaviours started creeping in around this time, too. One of the offshoots of having a racing mind and/or chronic anxiety was that sleep had always been a stranger to me. From the age of five I was terrified of the endless black and intrusive silence of the night. I would dread the moment when everybody went to bed, because that's when I knew it would just be me. This fear had followed me into adulthood and I never found a YouTube video containing the perfect life hack for sleep that worked when I needed it to. It turns out that eight pints of Guinness on an empty stomach would usually do the trick. The grogginess and foggy dehydration of the next day was a small price to pay for six hours of unconsciousness. However, all unhealthy things must come to an end and eventually even the sedative effects of alcohol stopped working. Which is the worst feeling in the world, by the way. Alcohol and insomnia are an awful combination. Lying in bed, staring at the ceiling, feeling the effects of the booze wear off and drain from your body, until you're lying limp, like a wounded animal, helpless and thirsty, furious with yourself for allowing this exact same scenario to have played out yet again. Fortunately (or unfortunately, as the nature of this book will reveal) it was around this time that I stumbled across Night Nurse, an over-the-counter cold and flu remedy that aids restful sleep. I realised fairly quickly that if I took a few swigs out of a bottle at the end of a night out, I'd definitely get some hours of rest. Now I know it's not exactly shooting meth on skid row, but it quickly became a nightly occurrence and soon I was swallowing half a bottle of the stuff before bed. A relatively concerning nightcap, if you ask me. One time, I remember downing an entire bottle and sleeping right through the following day until 8 p.m. I woke up and didn't know whether it was Tuesday or giraffe.

The heavy sessioning started to take its toll again. I was getting tired of feeling tired. My relationship with alcohol, just like my relationship with myself, was riddled with contradictions, though. Every time I took a break from booze and had a sense of life getting under control, I would go on a streak of self-destruction and create more problems for myself than I ever began with. And that worked both ways. If things ever got really bad, which they often did, I would always manage to step back from the ledge just in the nick of time and perform an emergency reset on my life. I remember one time going to my therapist when I finally ran out of steam – and money, probably – and we spent the entire hour exploring alternative high-adrenaline activities that I could participate in instead of drinking. If only there was a rehab for people who *sort of* fuck their lives up. I'd say it would be full. I certainly would have checked myself in very early on. Imagine a clinic for those who exist in the grey area, those who are definitely a bit fucked up, but because they've yet to fondle their own faeces on the back row of a bus, they're left to their own devices.

In the absence of such an institution, I developed my own little tool kit to deal with my drinking problem (it was only a *problem* back then, which meant it could be *solved*). This usually consisted of three or four weeks of sobriety to prove to myself that I wasn't an alcoholic, followed by one night of drinking, then two, then three ... until totally embracing the mayhem before I burned out and had to start the process all over again. Time would reveal this to be the fulcrum of all my problems – repeatedly doing the same thing and constantly expecting different results. This circle of strife. A hamster wheel of regret, repair and repeat. That big red 'fuck it' button, always at the tip of my finger, proved far too tempting not to touch and I spent most of my life stabbing it repeatedly. It made little to no sense. I could start the day in hiding, shunning the outside world and recoiling from humanity because I felt so low in myself; and spend that same evening prancing around nightclubs in a three-piece suit, high on life and embracing every person I vaguely knew. It sounds like mental illness, and part of the mania probably was. But mostly it was of the spiritual variety. I was at a point in my life when I was making the most money, living a life of material abundance, surrounded by countless 'friends', yet I was drowning in disconnection from self and speedily heading towards internal destruction. Again, it's very hard to pick up the phone and say to one of your mates 'Howiye, listen, I know things look great at the moment and everybody is congratulating me on building this business. And I know that I've been acting like I'm the dog's bollocks, eating in fancy restaurants midweek and spending absurd amounts of money, but I'm wondering if you've noticed that I seem a bit untethered from my soul?' When you play a part convincingly, very few people will ask questions. I've also learned in recovery that alcoholism is the 'disease of incomplete', and no amount of money or attention would ever make me feel enough. Make me feel whole. My heart belonged somewhere else. I just wasn't sure where yet. At this point, music was the only area of my life where I showed genuine glimpses into how I really felt, and who I really was. The career wasn't happening yet, but I was certain it would eventually. It was just a case of waiting for the phone to ring. One day soon, I knew I'd get a call from someone, somewhere, whisking me off to foreign lands to write songs and to pursue my dreams. In hindsight, I can see that this style of thinking was the stuff of sheer fantasy and only a seasoned madman might approach life like this.

But life is funny sometimes, and it mocks our attempts at understanding it, so you can only imagine my surprise when the phone *did* ring. And I *was* whisked away to foreign lands to write songs and pursue my dreams. I was given the opportunity to go over to New York with Markus Feehily (of Westlife) and to work on his solo album. It was a dream come true. I had met Mark several months before at a music festival and since then had been badgering him with demos and songs I was working on in my bedroom. We became friends. He was such an intensely kind person that I found it almost overwhelming. In the circles I moved in, sincerity was a rare commodity. The masculine, boisterous and intrinsically misogynistic social environments I had been in for most of my life had led to me confusing empathy with weakness (same-sex schools should be abolished, I think). Yet here was this superstar, with a musical ability I had never witnessed anything even close to, encouraging me to write honest music and 'be more like Mark'. He touched my life in a way that I wouldn't realise the impact of until years after we went our separate ways, and I will be forever indebted to him. I shouldn't be saying this as if he's dead, though. He's not. And this is not a eulogy. I'm still in touch with Mark today and he has a deservedly beautiful life. He is also still as endlessly supportive as one might imagine and would give the time of day to anybody.

In any case, between binges, I put down some lyrics on top of an instrumental that Mark had been sent by a producer. I wrote a quick chorus for a song that would later become 'Sirens' on his album. He loved it and we flew out to the US to work on the project and to take in the sights. We were quite the odd couple. Mark was really motivated and excited about working on the music. He had this weird trait of really caring about his work and valuing the time required to make good art. Meanwhile, all I really wanted was to go to bars in Manhattan and tell people that I'd flown out to New York to make music. I had received enough validation from the invitation to work on songs – now all I wanted to do was drink. In the end, it was a fun trip and we did manage to get some work done. I spent most of the week pissed and flew home to Dublin thinking I was Bernie Taupin. I remember meeting Harry Styles with Mark on a few of those nights, actually. This was back when One Direction were on the precipice of taking over America and becoming crazy megastars. Harry was very polite and endearingly starstruck when he met Mark from Westlife. When I was introduced to him my immediate thought was, 'Wow, this guy has a beguiling air about him, it's almost as if he could literally shag the entire universe.' And my second thought was, 'I wonder if he thinks the same about *me*?' Well, my friends, there are very few certainties in life, but I think we can all agree that death, taxes and the fact that Harry Styles has never once reflected on that encounter with me again are a guarantee.

By the time we got back to Dublin, I thought I'd outgrown the place. A week in New York can do that to you. The nightclub stuff had slowed down and I found myself low on cash, returning to the gilded limbo that is living at home in your mid-twenties, unsure of what to do next. The music stuff was moving along in the background, but it would be a while before Mark's album came out. I started to get the itch to create something again. Something new. Something different. These constant creative reinventions may be my Achilles heel, because they would completely alter my direction in life and the course of my 'career' – making it even harder to have a 'career' in the first place – but they're also what kept me going throughout times of existential despair. There is no cure to any woe of mine like the arrival of a new idea. The moment it lands out of thin air, when you least expect it, boom! The very room you are standing in looks completely different. It's as if the world is brand new. It's a different colour. It's a complete refresh. It's what keeps me alive, truthfully.

At this point, it's worth mentioning that in addition to my love for music, I have always been obsessed with comedy. With a gun to my head, if I could only choose one, it would come right down to the wire as to which has had a greater impact on my life. One of my earliest memories as a child was when my older brother stormed into the upstairs bathroom to find me standing on a stool, pulling different faces in the mirror. I always loved to entertain. Not to be confused of course with the memory of my teenage years when the same older brother would storm into the bathroom to find me masturbating with a J cloth. As I said, I *loved to entertain*.

Anyway, I was lying in bed one day and I had an idea for a character. Fortunately I didn't think about it too much and just started recording myself performing a monologue on my phone. The character was a deadpan version of myself and would reveal in dry, muted detail whatever issue he was facing that day. I would like to say there was more to it, or that it had been thoroughly planned, but that was not the case. I was simply lying in bed hungover and thought, 'Ah fuck it, I'll lash this up on Facebook.' Within half an hour the video had over 5,000 likes and shares. In today's era, where 'likes' can reach the 100,000s, that may not seem like a lot, but at the time it was stratospheric. Family members in England were even getting texts about it. From that day onward, a character was born and would mark the 'formal' beginning of my long and meandering relationship with the world of comedy.

Going viral is a bizarre thing to happen to anybody. You are catapulted from utter obscurity into a weird, fleeting and dysfunctional plane of selfies, heckles on the street and other bits of recognition. People know you but they don't know *how* they know you. And so they say that to your face. They look at you curiously, expecting you to answer. But *caveat emptor* – if you do hazard a guess as to how they might recognise you, they're immediately disappointed. The awareness of your own 'fame' that you've just shown instantly renders it null and void. Dull and unexotic. You're boring them now. You're not supposed to *know*, you see. They wanted to feel like they've discovered you and have cracked the code. Or worse, they conflate you with the character that you play on the internet, so when they say hello to you and you reply as yourself in the real world, they stare at you with intense disappointment, as if you've just told their first-born child that Santa is not real or that their parents are getting divorced. Alas, my first, brief snapshot of 'fame' was so minuscule on the Richter scale of celebrity that it would be absurd to even complain about it. And most of it is extremely flattering, let's be honest. It's very weird, but still flattering. I made the most of it. It was another excuse to show my face around the bars and clubs of Dublin, dining out on the occasional acknowledgement of a stranger or the lascivious glance from an excited Facebook follower in a nightclub.

Now, this next part may come as a shock to you, so perhaps you'd like to be seated. Earlier in the book, I spoke about the 'hole in the soul' and how from a very young age I never really felt complete. You've probably ascertained at this stage that my way of filling that void was to seek out fame, recognition and validation wherever I could. Perhaps if I devoured enough 'life', I would start to feel whole? Once I started going viral, I was certain that my internal unrest would be soothed. I was finally, properly getting the attention that I craved. People were messaging me every day telling me how much they loved my videos. I was being stopped in the supermarket. Not only that, but I was also schmoozing my way into the land of the celebrity, thanks to riding on Mark Feehily's coat-tails. This should be my moment – I would finally *arrive*.

But it wasn't. It wasn't like that at all. The effects of the heavy drinking had started showing, and I developed a type of social anxiety that I had never experienced before. I was nervous walking into rooms. I started experiencing panic attacks when meeting new people.

It got to the stage where I would sometimes circle a place for 15 or 20 minutes before going in. Oftentimes getting out of taxis on the way to places, feigning an illness and going home. In Los Angeles one time with Mark Feehily, I flatly refused to go to a few very important music meetings due to my 'nerves' getting the better of me. I would hyperventilate and suffer a complete panic attack, which would result in me needing to leave. Have you ever suffered from imposter syndrome and an ego complex at the exact same time? It's like you're caught between the feeling that you don't deserve to be in the place you're in, that you're not good enough; and you're also deeply angry at yourself for being crippled by that fear, because you know that it's preventing you from reaching your potential? On top of that, there are the resentments at just how naturally it seems to come to other people. After all that, I found myself, at 24, having the exact same problems that I had when I was 14, down by the riverbank. The only difference was that now I *needed* the alcohol. Right before my eyes, I could see the real power of choice disappearing in front of me. Now, I *had* to drink in order to walk into certain rooms. Not only that, but after experiencing the success of Brooklyn Zoo, creating viral Facebook videos and flying around the world with a pop star, I was faced with the panicked realisation that none of this was going to be enough.

MYTH:

Once I receive recognition for my work as an artist, I will settle down and enjoy life without excessive drinking.

REALITY:

My appetite for success in music and comedy ran parallel to my love for drinking. My biggest mistake was conflating the two or assuming that if I received validation in the eyes of others externally it would satisfy the internal, root urge to escape. I drank because I loved drinking. And I would always drink, regardless of the outcome of other aspects of my life.

I believed the lies I told myself. It was the greatest distraction I had ever known. I did the same thing in relationships. It's very easy, over a few glasses of wine, to ignore all the obvious problems and envision a future with the person sitting across from you. It dulls the voices of question. It reassures, comforts and helps frame the future in a softer, gentler light.

Although I may not have required a trip to rehab for my drinking yet, I was definitely losing sight of shore in terms of control. Alas, there wasn't any time for that. It would be much, much easier to play a different card. One that required not dealing with the issues. So that's exactly what I did. It was time to pull another *geographic*. The old reliable. An Irish exit from Ireland. Back to the cold, distant and anonymous embrace of the UK. It hadn't worked before, but surely this time would be different?

CHAPTER 4

LONDON FALLING

No matter where I went in the world, I would always bring my head with me.

I moved into a shed in East London in 2015. At the back of a house in Clapton, in Hackney. It was essentially a granny flat – if your granny went on Tinder dates and spent most of her pension on cans of Red Stripe. Of the many embarrassing habits that I nurtured throughout my years of drinking, I think smoking Pall Mall cigarettes while lying in bed in that airless cemented hut was the least acceptable. I was the South Dublin equivalent of Onslow from *Keeping Up Appearances*. Stubbing out my used butts in a makeshift ashtray – usually a half-empty glass of water – or absent-mindedly tapping the cigarette in the air, hoping the ash would land on the inside of a slipper on the floor. I probably didn't list *that* under the 'hobbies' section of my Bumble profile.

There were six people living in the house on Gunton Road that my shed was attached to, and we shared the same kitchen and living areas. A varied mix of DJs, reiki healers, plumbers and goths. It was your quintessential East London house-share and if there was a specific period in my life that I could time travel back to, this would be it. The others were from 'up north' – Leeds and Newcastle, mostly – and the dynamic between us worked instantly. Baker, Grainger, Matty H, James H, Stuart and Ruby. They were warm people, familiar and very, very funny. We were unified by the same two passions – music and comedy. David Brent and Daft Punk. Also worth mentioning that it's nearly impossible not to be reduced to a weak-kneed cooing lamb when hearing someone with a Yorkshire accent refer to you as 'kid'. It's homely and reassuring. Needless to say, they accepted me from the outset and we became good friends. We would get drunk together and have 'raves' in my shed, sometimes nearly 20 of us packed in like session sardines, sweaty and together, punching the roof with our fists and singing Kanye's 'Runaway', off our heads. Good times were had by everyone. It was normal, happy, run-of-the-mill partying, but at the same time it felt quite formative. I hadn't experienced that sense of a crew before, so it was nice to feel connected to a gang.

After those late nights of sessioning, we would spend the following morning in our local caff, talking shite and drinking watery tea. I'd pretend to have a passing interest in football while consuming sausages that would warrant a day in The Hague for anybody involved in making them and the lads would nip across to the bookies, placing various bets on the Scunthorpe versus Brentford match, or whatever latest football clash was on the TV that afternoon. In the evening, everybody would retire to their respective bedrooms, licking their wounds and dusting themselves off after a heavy weekend, with the looming thud of a Monday on the horizon. Meanwhile, I would retreat back into my shed with 12 cans of Red Stripe and a packet of Pall Mall from the corner shop, just to stave off the fear. I never wanted the party to end.

At first it was perfect. I was living in London, meeting various music publishers and hoping to sign a deal off the back of Mark Feehily's album, which came out around then. I had a little studio set up in the back of the shed and was making tunes every day. Rather than writing more pop songs, I started sampling eighties funk and bits of rare groove that I found on YouTube, making French-touch-inspired disco music. Things began to flow. I was inspired by the vibrancy of East London. In what would appear to be a classic case of 'fish-out-of-water Irishman is blown away by what happens in big cities', I was genuinely amazed by the size of London, the volume of artists there, the space there was for multiple genres and styles to exist at the same time, and the sheer number of different people devoting themselves to doing whatever it was they wanted to, creatively. The lack of convention, across the board, drew me in and inspired me. I got a buzz off the anonymity London provided, without realising then that that *same* anonymity would eventually swallow me whole. Every night there was a different gig, gallery launch or DJ set to go to. Someone to see or somewhere to go. I didn't need an excuse. Without making a conscious decision, I also slipped back into what seemed to be my UK routine of drinking by myself – but it felt okay this time, because *this time* I was happy. And it was quite normal among my English friends to go down the pub if you found yourself at a loose end, anyway. All in all, I had never been as stimulated in my entire life. I may have been playing the eternal waiting game that is wanting a career in the arts to take off – where the odds are never in your favour – but at least now I was part of a much bigger scene, where many people were chasing the same dream. I had a sense of community.

Bolstered by the intense support of my house-mates, I started sending my songs to labels and DJs I respected. Due to my brief bit of exposure to the world of mainstream pop music with Mark Feehily, I had always viewed myself as far too 'commercial' for any of the cooler electronic stuff to be taken seriously. I thought people would smell the 'Westlife' off me from a mile away. I say this as if I had won five Grammys, which obviously isn't the case, nor is the global stardom of Westlife anything to be sniffed at, but I guess I just felt a bit too mainstream for these electronic labels. In the end, I was wrong about that too. Thanks to the motivational kick up the arse I got from the lads, I threw the kitchen sink at making disco and things started to take shape. In September 2015, the Glaswegian DJ Jackmaster wanted to sign one of my tunes to the pioneering Scottish label Numbers. I had been a fan of Numbers for years and to release with them would be a dream come true. They put out music by the likes of Sophie, Hudson Mohawke and Kornél Kovács. Artists I truly admired. It was a very exciting time. In November, Jack included my tune 'I Need a Man' in his 2015 Mastermix, which was quite the hat tip, and it really felt like things were starting to happen. I usually loathe to use the word 'energy', but at this point in my life, it was there in abundance. I had momentum. I was finally *here*, in the right place, at just the right time. It would take an idiot to fuck this one up.

I then got into a relationship with someone who not only lived in the opposite side of London, but came from an entirely different world. We met through friends back home and within a few weeks of seeing each other, I moved out of the garden shed in Clapton into a two-storey penthouse in South Kensington. Intensity was my second language. I always thrived off spontaneity, even when it veered towards recklessness. When

I got to West London, in terms of being out of my depth, you might as well have dropped me into the hull of the *Titanic* with a snorkel and a pair of jelly shoes. At the time, I thought it was the right thing to do, of course. My little shed was way out east and the person I was seeing at the time came from a fortune so large that it would make my cushy Dublin suburban childhood seem like the meagre upbringing of a medieval serf. It seemed to make sense to move out west, to live rent-free and be a little bit more 'part' of life. Although I loved living out east, I felt a bit out on the fringes, and I was drawn towards the 'mainstream' trappings of West London, where many Irish people I knew were living at the time, that I had once avoided. Looking back, I was definitely swept up by the glamour of the whole thing, too. From the word go, I struggled with feelings of inferiority. I couldn't accept that I was *enough* just the way that I was and would thus spend the duration of our relationship feeling triggered and waiting to be told as much. We had an intense year that was saturated with turbulence. Just like in job interviews, the version of me I had sold her in the beginning differed greatly from the cracked and flawed real-life article that would present itself soon after. I'm sure that this is probably the case for many of us. You don't put your crazy in the shop window; you leave it in the back, hidden and out of the way. I did my best to act blasé, as if I, too, was a frequent flyer on private jets and totally familiar with the protocol of giving the food order to the chef the day before you fly, but it was a fool's errand. I just couldn't escape the realities of my own life – the fact that I struggled to pay for my Ryanair flights home for Christmas or that I'd recently failed a credit check when trying to switch my phone from credit to bill pay.

I was acting one way and feeling another. Plunged into a world that nobody expected me to understand yet for some insane reason I was obsessed with proving that I could belong.

I'm beginning to notice some consistency here ... Either way, it takes an awful lot of energy to appear nonchalant. I was becoming less like Onslow in *Keeping Up Appearances* and increasingly similar to Hyacinth herself. (I've been reassured that the resemblance to Mrs Bucket is only *marginally* physical.)

The intensity didn't end within the walls of my relationship. Moving to South Ken would herald the beginning of a new wave of 'outsiderness' that would ultimately generate catastrophic results. The smart thing to do would have been to turn on my heels and get myself back out to Hackney where I felt safe and that I belonged, but I was not in the business of doing smart things. I simply stayed put and tried to compensate for the unease by acting like this was all perfectly normal. Although I was usually quite au fait when it came to adapting to extremes, this was a very unique context, and I lost the run of myself fairly quickly. It's funny how effortlessly we can adjust to excess and how fast some novelties wear off.

Most notably, I remember one time in Mykonos awaiting the arrival of a private plane that was coming to pick us up, and feeling a genuine, intense disappointment when I realised that it wasn't the same size plane as the one we had flown over in. I literally thought to myself, 'You have well and truly lost it now, mate ... Also, where the hell is my sushi?'

It was a very strange chapter of my life and probably the dawn of me realising that no level of external luxury would satisfy my appetite to escape. I just wanted to get pissed, really. None of the other stuff actually meant as much to me. Everything had always felt a bit finite, anyway. Since the year before I sat the Leaving Cert, I really felt like my time was limited. When I was drinking, though, that's when everything felt alright. That summer I somehow ended up spending a week on a 90-metre superyacht, owned by a famous billionaire, and one night one of the most recognisable models on the planet came for dinner with her husband. I will always remember the moment when I was sitting across the table from her, a genuine icon, as she regaled the group with fascinating stories, and the only thing going through my head was 'Why is it taking so fucking long for that barefoot boat boy to refill my wine glass?' That was what I cared about. Nothing else mattered. I would have slept in the literal hull of the boat, down in the hold where they kept the jet skis, slurping seawater from one of my East London slippers if it meant that I could also drink as much wine as I wanted, uninterrupted.

I was quite good at hiding it, though, and for a while my drinking was just about fine. Among the peaks and valleys there were occasional plateaus. Brief stints of time where the wheels may not have been attached to the vehicle but they weren't entirely coming off either. My addiction was there, pretty visible if you went looking for it, but on a good day it might blur into the background of my identity, muddied by the boisterous persona and cigarette smoke. I was still the musician guy who did a bit of comedy and had a background in nightclubs, so it wasn't odd that I liked the odd pint. Anybody around me during these drinking 'plateaus' would probably argue that they didn't exist, but, internally at least, it's when things were okay. People enjoyed the flair I brought to the table, anyway. I was a *character* and a *bit of craic*. It was expected that I'd be slightly rough around the edges and to have a few unfit-for-the-dinner-table anecdotes. These fleeting interludes of not complete mayhem – usually arriving after a behemoth fuck-up, relationship breakdown or fresh start in a new city – would only ever last a couple of weeks, though. Chaos was always waiting just around the corner.

Back in London, I tried to fit in with the South Ken lot, but it was never going to work long term. Whether it was the linen shirts or the ketamine, I just couldn't find my flow or match their rhythm.

Everybody was called Rupert, Giles, Harry, Louis or Miles. To them, life seemed so relaxed and easy. I was bitterly jealous. I couldn't figure it out. There was a genuine *lightness* to extremely wealthy people that I could never understand, let alone emulate. I always had at least one or two internal and external fires on the go that required putting out. My administrative affairs were in a permanent state of disarray too, and there was an ever-growing pile of unopened envelopes, shoved into the back of my bedside locker, containing red warnings about unpaid bills, signed by a debt collector. Club nights were harder to operate and make a success of when working out of London, and my income was inconsistent and meagre. There is no worse feeling than chasing invoices for incredibly tiny sums but knowing that you depend on them. I developed an enormous inferiority complex as a result of feeling inadequate. I thought I was too coarse, too brash and, if the truth be told, too *Irish* for my girlfriend's friends and their public school-educated, softly spoken and gentle demeanours. All of it was in my head – most of them were actually very nice. And some of them were literally Irish, for fuck's sake!

Meanwhile, in music land, I had spent several months going back and forth with the Numbers crew up in Glasgow about my own release – deciding on the B sides, discussing artwork, etc. But it wasn't meant to be. In the end, there was a technical issue with the sample and the record didn't come out. I was devastated. It felt like a rejection from the world of music as a whole. Rather than viewing it as a temporary setback and still a positive indication that I could produce tunes at a high level, I saw it as the gates of my career closing. My emotions only dealt with extremes and after years of knocking on the door this was the worst possible outcome. It was the one thing I had in my back pocket when dealing with the imposter syndrome out West and when that happened, the arse fell out completely of my sense of self. I was properly beaten.

Ironically, it was only when the Numbers deal fell apart that I actually got offered and subsequently signed a publishing deal for my other songwriting work. It was with the Music Sales Group and provided a last-ditch, eleventh-hour, almost consolatory insulin hit of validation for my music career. It should have been a major milestone in my musical journey and it's one that

I will forever regret not embracing more vigor-
ously. The subsidiary label I signed to was called
Aim Low Music and it had an impressive roster of
artists beside whom I was honoured to be listed.
Acts like Tiger & Woods and Dean Blunt, artists
who made incredible music. Gone were the days
of big money advances in the music industry –
certainly for small-time songwriters like me – but
I did receive a modest bonus when I put pen to
paper. I should have used this as an incentive to
get back into the studio and to continue writing.

Instead, I decided to drink my way around
South West London, smiling in the face of its
unconquerable opulence, as if to say, 'See, I told
you I could do it.' Truth be told, I ran out of energy.
The drinking was sapping me of my ambition
and there had been too many knock-backs, and
I took every one of them straight to heart. For
far too long I had told my family and friends
that this next 'thing' was going to be *the* thing.
Conversations at Christmas were the worst, justi-
fying my career choices to relatives and friends,
swearing that the next project was going to be
the one that took me to the top. This would be
the gig, the meeting or the email that would act
as the flint which would then cause the spark

and my whole life would set alight in glory. I was sick of hearing myself saying it and I was even more sick of the excuses that I would then have to make when invariably it didn't happen. Painfully scanning the room, searching for the right thing to say while desperately trying to justify myself, hiding behind a glass of red wine and doing my best to ignore that look on people's faces, eyebrows raised with a half-jaded, almost wry, 'Sure, I could have told you that ages ago' smile painted on their faces. And yes, maybe they could have told me that. But why share inspirational quotes on your Instagram page about failure being a natural ingredient of success if you're not going to practise what you preach and encourage those around you to pursue their dreams?

I think the most embarrassing element of failure that I struggled with was the feeling of self-centeredness. I was mortified for trying in the first place. I could have been spending my life doing anything more virtuous, yet here I was approaching the latter end of my twenties, still determined to receive recognition for my own creative work. It felt like an absurdly arrogant way to spend your life, trying to convince the world that you're brilliant. The line between self-expression and self-obsession felt very thin at times. It still does. I often wondered if I would have been better off pursuing a more conventional career, but I just didn't know how to do anything else. The dice had already been rolled. Most importantly, the closest I ever came to a primal sense of purpose or feeling like I belonged anywhere was when I was making music or writing comedy. Most other things left me unfulfilled and a bit sad.

With the Numbers deal gone and a lost sense of momentum, I started to feel very low in myself. The abject misery of wandering around West London during the day, surrounded by some of the wealthiest people on the planet, while struggling to figure out what my own basic purpose was, really began to really take its toll. I started handing my CV into TV production companies and creative agencies, desperate to escape the sorrow of my collapsed dreams in music by rustling up a career in TV or something in the comedy world. I had created viral marketing campaigns when working in the nightclub world, so I just assumed I would be a shoe-in for a nine-to-five in any modern work environment. It turns out 'drinking pints' doesn't actually qualify as a valid answer when an interviewer asks you how you spent the previous seven years and to comment on your experiences. I still cringe with embarrassment when I think about the time I went for an interview as an events co-ordinator for a wine delivery company based in Bermondsey. I thought that I'd nailed the interview and went out for a few beers that afternoon to celebrate. At around 7 p.m., I received a very kind email saying, 'Thank you for your time today, Mark. Unfortunately, we don't think you're right for this role, but we wish you the best of luck with the job search.' In my mortifying drunken wisdom, I thought it would be a good idea to reply immediately with 'hahahahahahah you can shove your job up your holes, I didn't even want it in the first place'. Good stuff. I'll probably lose sleep tonight, now that I've dislodged that memory from the unknown location my brain had buried it, deep within the crevices of my soul.

The job hunt was yielding little in the way of results and beginning to eat away at my optimism. Idleness is the enemy of the soul, after all. My way of dealing with this expanding inferiority complex, coupled with a sense of artistic defeat and generalised malcontent, was to drink myself into a stupor on nights out, until I was comfortable enough to occupy the same space as the people I deemed myself beneath. I started getting sloppy.

MYTH:

When I was drunk, I could hold my own and outwit even the most Etonian of wankers in Chelsea.

REALITY:

I was just a bit of a disaster. My interpretation of 'holding my own' usually meant arguing with confused and uninterested bystanders, who brushed past me slightly aggressively in the queue for the bar.

When introduced to friends of my girlfriend, I would immediately act standoffish and adopt a defensive disposition, until later on when I was nearly cross-eyed and would search for things to argue about with her or anybody else at the table. It's as if I wanted an opportunity to prove that I could hold my own, that I was good enough, and my drunken-minded way of doing this was by starting and then attempting to win an argument. It wasn't exclusive to friends either. Whether it was the Hereford Arms, the Phene, the Sydney or the Duke of Clarence, there were several times people had to pull me out of pubs after an argument with a stranger that had stemmed from my outrage at some perceived slight. I was bitter and aggressive. It became harder to walk when wearing the weight of all the chips on my shoulder.

My girlfriend eventually had the courage to call my behaviour out for what it was. This led to the watershed moment when I would first hear the dreaded two-word combo 'your' and 'drinking'. The alcoholic's worst nightmare. 'Mark, we need to talk about your drinking.' 'My drinking?' I still recall the mock surprise. Nothing prepares you for the deep shame and outrage of hearing that accusation for the first time. You've been waiting for it for a long time, but it still stings when it meets your ears. At this stage, I knew that my relationship with alcohol was a destructive one, but I sort of thought that it was *my* secret, and I was probably still under the illusion that the issues caused by my drinking were mostly just a reaction to the external rather than an extension of the root problem. I presumed that I was merely a sensitive guy, with a very busy mind, and when I had a lot going on, I turned to alcohol a little more than your average person. I wasn't sneaking sips at breakfast time or forcing down mouthfuls of Dettol just to catch a buzz. Once life sorted itself out, surely my drinking would too? 'Mark, we need to talk about your drinking.' I will never forget it. It's strange, too, because there was definitely a part of me that wanted to feel the release of defeat and accept help from the hands that were clearly reaching out to me, but that would be giving in, and I wasn't quite ready for that yet. Instead I let my ego get in the way of potential happiness and responded only with anger and blame. You could have called me any insult under the sun and I would barely have batted an eyelid, but being accused of being an alcoholic? Game over. My best thinking told me that the perfect way to deal with an accusation like this was to go out on the piss, of course. If anything, just to prove how wrong she was. Nine pints of Estrella and a few abusive text messages would show my ex-girlfriend how stable I was. 'My drinking? How dare you? Were you not drinking too over the last few days? I wasn't even doing drugs, half the people there were off their heads on bag, what do you mean, my drinking, ~~you stupid fucking bitch~~?' And that is the version of the text message that has likely been sanitised by my memory. But it was too late. I had been seen. Even in rooms where everybody else was drinking, I was drinking differently. My 'why' was not the same as theirs and you could see it on my face. I was in a bad place.

Things quickly began to deteriorate. My relationship with booze had always been in tandem with the one I had with myself – so when one engine failed, the other followed suit. I was sick of the person I was becoming and I knew that I needed to make a great change in my life. It was make or break. The drinking had finally taken centre stage and it was starting to affect my relationships and my career. It was all well and good when I was living in the blissful obscurity of my little East London shed, just out of harm's way, and hand-picking who I saw, when I saw them and how I saw them. But under the glaring, surgical lights of real life, where one is expected to manage relationships, to socialise as a part of wider groups and generally *be okay*, I would always be found out. I could only spin the plates for so long. I wasn't able to just get along in the way other people did. I developed a familiar feeling that there was a clock ticking. It wasn't a new sensation.

Truth be told, I had felt like there was a clock ticking since the day that I was born; I was always waiting to be pulled aside and quietly told that I was doing life wrong and needed to re-read the instructions.

But this time it was bad. I knew that living life like this wasn't sustainable and something had to give. I used to joke with my therapist about how my drinking was a problem and one day I would have to call it quits and check myself in somewhere. I stopped making these jokes. It was becoming too real. There was a deeper, creeping unease in my stomach that I first felt in Brighton, but now it was back and it was an awful lot heavier. It was as if the alcohol was turning on me and my defence against it wasn't the Fort Knox I once thought it was. The one thing that took me away from reality and far away from myself was now only adding things to the list of problems I had whenever I woke up. I hated myself for becoming an angry drunk, for making a fool of myself on nights out, for always saying the wrong thing, for lying to people, for causing problems, for being mean to my girl-friend, for sending crazy messages, but I couldn't seem to stop. Truthfully, I didn't even want to. I just wanted things to be different, and to learn how to drink better. Maybe it was the spirits. Or actually, maybe it was the beer. I shouldn't drink on an empty stomach. Or midweek. I had to figure it out. I couldn't understand how every-body else managed to get drunk and not want to start crying.

The time had come to do something drastic and I knew I had to do it fast. My relationship had fallen apart, my career was non-existent and my self-esteem was on the floor. I was tired of all the extremes. From living 'the life' in Los Angeles to going straight back to my mother's couch. From selling DVDs in Brighton just to buy a few cans, to sleeping with several thousand euro under my bed every night in the heyday of Brooklyn Zoo. It had gone on way too long. The only constant in my life up until the age of 25 had been extremes. There was never any in between. My second language was chaos. But it wasn't working any more. I wanted to be steady and reliable. I wanted

to get off the train. It was time to stop. I wanted
to be normal.

And then I discovered cocaine.

CHAPTER 5

UNHAPPY ENDINGS

The first time I did a 'proper' drug was when a friend of mine sprinkled a bit of MDMA into my drink in a nauseatingly ironic Alpine-themed nightclub on Kensington High Street called Bodo's Schloss. If you transferred all of the music they played that night onto a USB stick and left it inside a time capsule for future civilisations to get a better understanding of us, their first reaction would almost certainly be 'Oh right, so they were wankers.' The drug took effect and all my anxieties evaporated. I loved the world around me and I tapped my feet to the sound of my seatbelt in the taxi on the way home. Then I woke up the next day and I wanted to kill myself. I couldn't deal with the comedown at all. It lasted about a week and was as if I was viewing the world in black and white. I don't think I was supposed to go that high. All the joy was sapped from my body and it was as if my brain was incapable of producing any emotion other than empty, tearful dread. It was a different type of sadness from the kinds I'd known before. It was even different from the iterations of nothingness that I also had a bit of form with. I was left with little more than a hollow voice and a racing mind. And it went on for what seemed like an eternity. Every day I would wake up, expecting it to have lifted, only to recede back further into my mind upon realising that it was *still there*. My friends talked about comedowns but this couldn't be that. Ten days in and I was still reeling. I went for a walk along the Thames one night and contemplated the worst. Right by Battersea Bridge. It was dark and I didn't want to face another night of staring at the ceiling. I was scared. The intrusive thoughts had become deafening. In the end I just got myself a kebab and went home, and I never told anybody about it. I was embarrassed at how dark my thoughts had become and I was angry at myself for not being better at controlling them. For a while afterwards, I steered clear of all *extracurriculars*.

Aside from that MDMA encounter, I was quite wet behind the ears when it came to drugs. I had smoked weed once when I was around 12, in my back garden with my older brother and his friends, but it didn't really do anything for me. After that, I didn't try it again properly until I was about 14, when I hit my first 'waterfall'. That time, I got so unbelievably stoned that I could only walk backwards and experienced a series of panic attacks alongside a bout of paranoia so bad that part of me *still* thinks the FBI are looking through my bins. The high from weed or hash just never really suited me. It didn't manifest in lazy days of Dorito-stained fingertips and nineties trash TV like I thought it would. I wanted a substance that would shift my perspective outwards rather than inwards. Weed simply amplified the internal cacophony of unease, but I was searching for something to silence it.

Aside from those brief skirmishes with other substances, I remained steadfast in my commitment to be drug-free. It became one of my fun facts, actually. A novel little titbit, a sort of *Did you know?* that I would whip out on Bumble dates after three bottles of rosé, along with the fact that I didn't have any tattoos or had never experienced a wet dream. I thought it made me interesting; that I could drink the way I did yet never go near the stronger stuff. Drugs were still about, though. Cocaine hadn't quite reached the ubiquity it has now – when it's snorted every weekend by most people with a beating heart and a working set of nostrils – but it was definitely on the scene. I didn't see the appeal. My first glimpse into what happens to my brain during a chemical comedown had done enough to scare me straight for quite a while. I knew that my head wasn't in a good place from all the boozing and I was cautious enough not to tempt fate any further. By sticking with alcohol, at least I had the perception of control. Anything stronger and it simply wasn't worth taking the risk.

But then again, what's the worst that could happen? As the relationship with my long-suffering girlfriend in West London was circling the drain, I started harbouring the insane idea that perhaps I was only getting so drunk all the time because I *wasn't* doing drugs. Exploring various ways to continue to drink was much more attractive than stopping drinking entirely. Maybe the odd line would straighten me out and make the nights out less problematic?

We were in Hammersmith one afternoon, about 20 of us, and everybody was getting stuck into the bag. It was only two o'clock and I was already four or five pints deep. I knew that if I kept going at my current rate, I would be legless by dinner and everybody else would only be getting started. I was tired of being the drunk guy, the guy who always seemed to have a problem with someone else at the table, the intense one who argued with his girlfriend in public and carried a general air of slop about him wherever he went. My perceived superpower of being able to drink for hours on end without being affected by the volume of beer inside me had disappeared entirely. My constitution was not what it used to be. Truthfully, part of me was now also curious to see what the cocaine high might feel like. Psychologically, I thought I had come to know most feelings, the good and the bad, the high and the low, and was interested in the idea of experiencing a *broader* mental shift and perhaps gaining a different perspective on life. I had been reassured by fellow panic attack sufferers that it wouldn't interfere with anxiety at all – they were wrong – and that cocaine simply makes you a little bit chattier and sharper, enabling you to drink more. They were sort of right with that part but still, mostly, very wrong. Either way, I was ready to join the party.

MYTH:

I will radiate enigmatic, chic sophistication when I finally decide to join the cocaine club.

REALITY:

Snorting a line for the first time turned out to be about as glamorous as a dose of scabies.

Back in Hammersmith, I was chaperoned to the bathroom by two of my friends, and we piled into a cubicle, exchanging whispers over keys. I was then given the instructions. I didn't snort the first bit properly and it ended up just falling back out of my nose, so I was completely covered in it, resembling someone who'd been shot in the face with Homer Simpson's make-up gun. The second time I did it right and fuck me, it burned. Almost like when you bend your head backwards in a swimming pool and the water goes up your nostrils, right into your sinuses. Aside from that I didn't feel anything.

Doing coke for the first time is sort of like losing your virginity. It never happens the way you thought it would. It's never in the place you imagined it would be either. It's definitely not like in the movies. It's crude and visceral. Familiar and underwhelming. It's like a slightly uglier and more mundane version of what you expected. Just like the first time I drank. Alcohol didn't taste as refreshing as it looked on television or in the hands of adults. It was just so bloody ordinary compared to what my brain told me it would be like. Not dissimilar to that jumper you bought online recently or the first five minutes of every single Tinder date. With cocaine, it all happens too quickly and there's something unmistakably dirty about it, with a constant underlying feeling of 'Is this *it*? Is *this* the thing that I've been warned about for all these years?' How many Tony Montana posters did I stare at on teenage boys' bedroom walls – when I was also a teenager, by the way – imagining what that mysterious white powder must feel like, only for this to be the flat reality. It didn't alter my mind in the way I thought it would. I could still get the stench of the urinals through my burning nostrils. I was still cramped into a filthy cubicle with puddles of piss on the floor in a pub near a train station. I was still *me*. It was about as sexy as a diagnosis of mumps. It doesn't really feel like you've taken anything, either. I thought the high would be instant and explosive, but it wasn't like that at all. It was all a bit ... meh. However, I will admit that I did have a sense of maturity after doing it. Almost as if I was a proper adult now. There was a temporary sense of feeling part of a club and one of the gang.

When we were finished with the formalities, I walked out of the bathroom feeling like I was a character in a movie. I definitely didn't feel like that on the night I lost my virginity, unless Michael Bay is planning on making a 37-second feature film. Good luck finding a 16-year-old body double who looks like Hyacinth Bucket, Michael.

After that disappointing foray into cocaine use, I knew that it wasn't my type of drug. Ultimately, it did nothing to enhance my enjoyment of the evening and judging by the *sent messages* folder on my phone, I was still just as sloppy and chaotic when under the influence of cocaine as I was when I was drinking. It didn't make sense to do any more of it.

So I started doing more of it. Every week, just to make sure that I knew what all the fuss was about, and eventually it began to grow on me. I could happily go without it, of course, I just *chose* not to. I wasn't concerned about the amount that I was doing, because I adhered to the many unspoken rules that I had when it came to cocaine use. Here are a few of them:

1. Always surround yourself with at least one person who does much more than you. Use them as your measuring tool. Find yourself a cosy spot in the middle of the group, above the ones who never do it and just below the people who always do it, even before they've had a pint. That's the sweet spot.
2. Don't be the person who suggests making the call/order.
3. Never be the one to meet the dealer.
4. Try not to pay for it.
5. Only do it when you drink.
6. Put up a faux fight – say 'Ah no, we won't' for at least 20 minutes before eventually agreeing to get the bag.

I was fascinated by the risk of becoming addicted to cocaine. I often wondered how that would feel, to be physically hooked on something. I'm aware now how stupid and absurd it was to be curious about what it might feel like to be addicted to something when I was drinking five times a week and smoking over 30 cigarettes a day. Movies told me that cocaine addiction was crazed, compulsive and completely manic in the way that it manifested. I found that confusing. None of the cocaine users I knew looked like the ones in the movies. They were almost all completely functional. I was conditioned to expect extremes and if it didn't get to that stage, well, then, it couldn't be addiction.

In my experience, lots of people who do cocaine think they are the exception to the rule. That was certainly my problem, anyway. I firmly believed that the way that I did it was different from the way anybody else did it. It wasn't as bad, I was slightly more *mindful*. In the end, my use *was* very unique and different from the way my friends used, but for all the wrong reasons. Most of the people I knew who were dabbling in the occasional line didn't sit in their bedroom alone on Sunday nights, working their way through their third bottle of red wine, before getting down on their hands and knees and swiping their fingers along the inside corners of their desk drawers, on the slight chance there might be enough cocaine residue to make their gums go numb.

It would take a good few months of dabbling, experimenting and 'Ah sure, only if it's going' before I realised that I couldn't stop doing it, even if I wanted to.

It was good craic, though, for a while at least. And in the beginning, I have to admit that it ameliorated my sense of *outsiderness* from the world around me. For a while, it made me feel like I belonged, like I was equal. Even now, I'm experiencing a slight euphoric recall, thinking about the very moment that I would slide my hand into the inside of my jacket on the way to the bathroom in a bar. The instant sense of safety from feeling the plastic edges of the tiny little bag brushing against your fingertips. *Nirvana*. It's there. The security of this sensation is almost childlike. It's akin to getting carried inside the house in your parent's arms as a child, after falling asleep during a long car journey. Nothing can disturb you in this place. Milliseconds before the hand goes into the jacket, there would always be an instinctive fear that the bag might be gone. Maybe it slipped out? Maybe it was stolen? But then you touch it and the relief washes over you. It's like a winning lottery ticket. *Let's go!* Everything, absolutely everything is going to be fine now and I am certain of it. Even the motion of the key first plunging into the bag is so smooth. There's just so much of it! It doesn't even touch the sides, just slides deep into the pure and endless white. There's no scraping required yet. For the first few trips, it's painless. This sharp-edged little metallic key works as the ladle to serve up the wholesome, celestial goodness. *Honey, I'm home.* It doesn't have to be a solo pursuit, either. There is a connection unlike any other, when you're huddled in a bathroom cubicle with a stranger or a friend, whispering intimately and sharing the secrets that you usually hide from yourself, over the passing of a car key, credit card or two-euro coin. It feels sacred. It feels everlasting. The relationship of a lifetime shoe-horned into five fleeting minutes. Until it's time to perform the final but vital routine of checking each other's nostrils, deciding who will go out first – as if that matters – and pretending to be talking about something mundane like your problems in life. Then, one last glance in the mirror, a quick look at your nose again, this time from the side, before turning to ask your new best friend and business partner, 'Are you sure I'm okay?', but he's already gone.

Once I began using cocaine, the effects on my temperament became visible immediately. I started behaving in ways that were at odds with my character. It wasn't just when I was drunk or high, either. My hangovers had evolved from slightly inconvenient little headaches into fully fledged miniature nervous breakdowns and oftentimes it wasn't until the next day when it became clear how fucked my thinking was. I couldn't handle the comedown. Those hangovers were emotional sagas. Monstrous, three-day affairs. It would take nearly a week for my moods to even semi-regulate. But by then it would be Thursday, and I'd be back on it again. The first sober evening after a binge was always the worst. Not the morning, because the booze would still be in my system then, sometimes even giving me a false sense of freedom, as if I'd got away with it. I'd grow confident, amazed at how okay I felt and delighting in the fact that I was walking away unscathed from a three- or four-day bender. Alas, 4 p.m. would eventually descend and with it, so would I. One minute I'd be trembling with fear, afraid to look at text messages, and the next moment I'd be smashing my phone into pieces in a rage. I couldn't sit still. No amount of leg-tapping, or playing with something in my hands, would ease the fearful energy coursing through my veins. I used to surprise and disgust people with my ability to smoke cigarettes when I was hungover. After a heavy few days of sessioning, I could easily smoke 40 on the first sober day, trying to catch my nerves. I inhaled cigarettes with such a speed and intensity that people would regularly ask me, 'Are you alright, Mark?' when I was in the middle of a drag. The partying was really starting to do a number on me. For about five years I was constantly on the verge of bursting into tears. There was always a breakdown of unholy propor-tions lurking right beneath the surface. I was erratic and itchy on my feet.

Naturally, I wasn't exactly the picture of emotional health when I was high, either. I went through all of the run-of-the-mill displays of deteriorating mental health, like punching holes in walls and leaping out of moving taxis, but there were also more concerning aspects. I remember one night I ordered a pizza after a three-day coke binge when I'd barely eaten a thing. For whatever reason, I became convinced that the delivery driver was intent on harming me, so I placed a fork in the pocket of my dressing gown and waited outside the front door by the green bin, planning to ambush him when he arrived. Fortunately, he decided not to deliver the pizza after being subjected to a drunken tirade over the phone, and he spared us both the indignity of him kicking the shite out of me in my dressing gown before calling the police and having me arrested. My girlfriend at the time was away and I have never told anybody that story until today. Cocaine is fucking mental.

My relationship finally ended a few months later, partly due to incompatibility and partly due to my drinking. I always prided myself on my ability to shake people off and move on as if they were nothing. But as soon as I found myself single again, free from the clutches of a relationship, I collapsed into a three-week bender that would take me from massage parlours on Wardour Street to Albanian drug dens out west – with a few All Bar Ones and Soho Houses thrown in for good measure. I never actually got a massage, either. I went in once with a friend of mine who wanted to get a 'massage' but I couldn't bring myself to find the situation sexual or to stop making jokes. I ended up paying the full price and then having to just sit in the lobby like a scolded child waiting outside the principal's office, while my friend received his paid-for relief. The woman behind the counter would look over her glasses every now and then, audibly tutting, as if to say, 'Pathetic'. She was dead right. A similar thing had happened out in Los Angeles a few years before, when I had dragged my friends to a strip club on Sunset Boulevard. I paid for a private dance but ended up just chatting to a stripper in this weird little booth, asking her about her hopes and dreams. I am a criminally embarrassing cliché at times. She wasn't too fussed about having a chat and mostly said things like, 'Hey, sweetie, why don't you try to relax and just focus on my titties?' I still remember how she said it. It was just like in the movies. *Mah tidd-eez.* I wanted to feel like Christian Slater in *True Romance.* Alas, even in a situation which had been a fantasy of mine since I was 14, I was still fantasising about it being different from how it was. All of this was irrelevant anyway – I'm pretty sure that as a successful stripper on Sunset Boulevard, this woman did not need my money, my pity or to be airlifted from her life by a 21-year-old peach-bodied alcoholic from Foxrock.

After the relationship ended, it quickly got grim in London. I was sleeping on friends' couches and drinking a lot by myself. Many a night I would find myself hovering outside the front of the Toucan in Soho, chasing a sense of belonging in other Irish people, before making conversation with someone I had nothing in common with, like a recruiter from Cardiff called Eddie, who had come to London for the night, and was just trying to enjoy a couple of quiet pints before going back to his hotel room. I'd deliver my usual bit of showmanship and charm, which would be enough to keep him enthralled and lead to Eddie and myself having a skinful together, with me dodging his questions about how I ended up drinking there by myself and reassuring him that my friends were on the way. My friends were always *on the way*.

Eventually I gave in and got the ferry back to Dublin with a friend. It was time to get out of Dodge again. Back to the drawing board. I suspect my parents' sympathy was beginning to wane due to the seemingly never-ending jumps back and forth across the Irish Sea, but they always welcomed me with open arms. Home would offer me the space to re-evaluate.

Comedy was where I saw my future but I had absolutely no idea about how to get there. Aside from the viral Facebook videos, I was also writing longer scripts and kept a notebook with hundreds of ideas that I would update daily. It didn't pay the bills, though. I was too early for the era of paid partnerships on social media and the most I ever got in exchange for my social media presence back then was a free pint. (Any money would have gone on pints anyway, though, so I suppose it's fair enough.) I was broke and I needed a 'real' job immediately. I couldn't afford to stay in London and conduct the search without a fixed abode or income. I was back in Ireland and determined to return to the UK as quickly as possible, to prove all of *them* wrong. My latest set of problems was the result of other people's personal shortcomings, as far as I was concerned. It was the sneering preppy public school boys from Chelsea that were the problem, not me ... the sneering, preppy, private school boy from Ireland. Or my drinking. Or my drug use.

That trip home on the ferry was a treacherous

one. It came off the back of a five-day bender with an old friend – who shall remain nameless – and myself and Keith were reckless beyond measure. After taking the two trains from London to Holyhead, where we dutifully drank for the duration, there were delays in the ferry times as a result of the weather, so we had about six hours to kill before the ship left. Now, I'm sure that the rest of Holyhead is absolutely stunning, but the particular pub we ended up in should be plastered on the side of every single bus in the UK and used as an example of where drinking could bring you. Grim isn't the word. Needless to say we drank in that pub for six hours and nearly missed the ferry. We arrived in the queue for security just in time, only for my friend to remind me that we had a decent bit of cocaine on our person. (Train cocaine, as we had *hilariously* nicknamed it.) One lost game of rock, paper, scissors later and I was opening the stitching in the back of my North Face jacket to place these three bags of coke inside the seam. Like a degenerate version of Daniel Day-Lewis in *Phantom Thread*. To this day, it was one of the most terrifying moments of my life. I remember thinking, 'You've wanted a career in comedy for how long and yet the first time you're going to appear on TV will probably be in a documentary presented by Michaella McCollum titled *The Holyhead Handover* or something equally woeful'. For the record, it wasn't *that* much cocaine. But as someone who had previously existed in a world of not smuggling *any* cocaine across borders, even our couple of measly bags seemed like a heavy shipment. As we approached the top of the queue, myself and my friend got pulled aside to be searched by security at the gate. I think it was a member of the Gardaí. At that moment, I knew that something was going to have to give. The way I was living my life was simply not sustainable. I started making promises to myself. This would be my reckoning. This would be the moment it all changes. I swore it. After patting me down with the vigour of a deeply dehydrated pensioner swatting a fly, the security man waved me through. We celebrated by going out on the upper deck of the boat and doing bumps off our fists. I cringe now at the insanity of it all.

Once back in Ireland, I maintained my new London hobby. I tried to stop on a few occasions, but it would always creep back in. The problem was that once I started drinking I would find myself thinking about it, whether I wanted to or not. Like a missed call from your ex or the minor criticism of a family member, it gets inside your head. I managed to keep it somewhat at bay. Two or three nights a week, usually. If I was with people who weren't on the bag, I would just rub it into my gums for the first half of the night, as an act of courteous restraint. Family gatherings or quieter nights with friends midweek. I felt like I was doing them a solid by not snorting full lines until it was at least 10 p.m. and sure by then, everybody was drunk anyway. I remember one night sitting in Searsons on Baggot Street with a good friend. I think it was a Tuesday. We'd walked over for a couple of pints after attending a charity table quiz for a local sports team. When ordering the two pints of Guinness from the waitress, I politely asked her if she had a number for some good cocaine in the area. My friend apologised profusely on my behalf and spent the rest of the evening trying to explain to me just how insane that was and did I need some sort of intervention. I still cringe when I recall my response: 'But in *London* ...'

Life became a bit of a slog. I was applying for jobs back in the UK, sending hundreds of emails a day, with the manic determination only

ever exerted by a man fresh out of a relationship, intent on proving to his ex that he's doing
perfectly fine without her. It's quite the rocket fuel,
as it turns out. Not to be confused with the other
rocket fuel that I was also partaking of, of course.
Things were shite but at the same time, I was
familiar with these intervals in life. Just another
unwanted hiatus due to my career choices. I was
an *artiste* after all, I was a comedian. Soon things
would pick up. This was just a little slow period.
Once the career happened, I would be fine. I
wasn't dry snorting. I wasn't staying up for three
days at a time. I was *grand*. Everybody was doing
it now, too. All the guys I'd known for years who
said they'd never go near it were all going near
it. My drinking was still a bit of a worry, but that
was just London, *mate*. I was now of the opinion
that alcohol and cocaine were maybe just part
of life. Like bad weather and traffic. Sure, I
might be a heavy drinker. But most artists were
heavy drinkers. I didn't need to act on any of the
concerns expressed by my ex-girlfriend and I
certainly didn't need to dig up old internal graves
where I knew something was terribly dysfunctional about the way I drank. I assumed my drug
use would just come to a natural ending, like a

holiday romance or outrage on the internet.

After six weeks in Dublin, I was going stir crazy. I couldn't deal with the manic highs of the weekend binges followed by the engulfing silence of the suburbs from Monday to Friday. I desperately needed to get back to London. Eventually, a plan was formed. I managed to get a temporary bed in the spare room of a friend of my mother's, who had repeatedly come to my rescue throughout the various break-ups and breakdowns of my chequered London career to date; and, most important, I got a job. I was to be the *managing director* of an electronic robot costume company based out in Brentford ... Your guess is as good as mine, to be honest. To this day, I don't know how I got that job. I also feel enormous guilt for the people in the company whose time I wasted. I'm fairly sure I concocted a spiel about spending my childhood watching *Robot Wars* and then developing a commercial interest in robots due to my cousin working as a set designer on *Interstellar*. Or something equally insane and untrue. I shouldn't have taken the job, I shouldn't have gone back to London. It happened at a point when I was well and truly descending into full-blown cocaine dependency and the chances of me sitting still in the job long enough for it to be fruitful were minuscule.

I went out drinking on the very first day I started the new position and showed up four hours late for work the following morning. I told them my Australian housemate had flooded the kitchen. In lieu of getting a qualified plumber to look at the fictional leak, they'd obviously called upon Mehigan to mop up the whole mess. There's an ironic metaphor in there somewhere. At the time, I felt secure in the lie by providing the nationality of my fake housemate who caused the fake leak, as it was more specific and thus more plausible. Within a few weeks, I was pulled aside and questioned in a very polite, considerate and respectful manner as to whether or not I had some issues with 'partying'. Once again, a hand offering help was stretched out in front of me. So I did what anybody in need of help would do, and I told him absolutely not. My fatal flaw, forever rearing its head, was the crippling inability to accept my own weakness and to ask for help in learning how to deal with them, or even take hold of the hand when it reached out to catch me.

In an effort to keep up appearances and

maintain the illusion that things were on the up, I had found myself a flat in Chelsea. Let me rephrase that – I had found a single bed in a tiny room on the top floor of a five-person flat-share on Finborough Road in Chelsea. Over the course of the next two months, I reverted to my old ways and my lifestyle quickly caught up with me. The job didn't work out and I decided to leave just shy of my three-month probation period. There are one hundred reasons I would have told people back then as to why I quit, but in reality, there was only one – I couldn't keep all the plates spinning. My drinking was interfering with my ability to get up for work in the mornings. I didn't enjoy the work I was doing or where I felt my life was heading, and the only way I knew how to deal with those feelings was to drink. I was dwindling, and fast.

Within six months, I was back in Dublin again, flat on my back. Of course the job didn't work out. Of course the flat didn't work out. It was all a disaster. I was a disaster. I had absolutely no idea what I was doing. My friend Kate had acted as my personal therapist for those six months, wrestling me back from the edge every time I came close to total destruction, but if nothing changes, *nothing* changes. Once again the wheels had come off. I came back to Ireland yet again, this time with even more chaos behind me and very little in front of me, other than a desire to work in comedy. It's all I wanted to do. My head was fried and I knew that I was running out of road. I just needed a break, the right opportunity, and the rest would fall into place.

And then I got a job in BBC Comedy.

CHAPTER 6

I MADE THE BBC!

With one final roll of the dice and in a giant leap towards legitimacy, I flew back to London to start working at the BBC. I fervently maintained the myth that if I had a job in a reputable organisation like the BBC, my drinking would iron itself out. Life would get in the way of the chaos. The reality turned out to be nothing remotely like that. Drinking would always get in the way of life.

When I arrived, I spent the first few weeks surveilling SpareRoom.co.uk in a ceaseless search to find a flat within my budget that would hopefully have fewer people living there than I had fingers. Seemingly undeterred by my previous scrapes with the Borough of Kensington and Chelsea, I sought out a place in neighbouring Fulham, a mostly bougie area that was slightly more expensive than I could afford, thus making it very desirable, and close enough to central London to instil the sense in me that I was moving on up in the world. Fulham wasn't dissimilar from South Dublin in many ways, and the sea of gilets, dachshunds and arseholes in every beer garden made it seem like a safe enough place for me to swim. I sought comfort in the familiar – it beat the fear of the unknown. The little abode I eventually found on Seagrave Road was advertised as a cosy home, where the successful applicant would be living with 'Two quiet working professionals, both in their late twenties, who enjoy the odd night out but mostly appreciate chilled evenings on the couch, watching *Game of Thrones* and eating a bit of choco after ordering a Deliveroo!' 'That's me!', I thought. '*I* like the odd night out on the town and *I* like Deliveroo. *I'm* cosy!' I was there a fortnight before I deemed them both to be uninteresting nerds and received my first written warning from the landlord for bringing people back for parties, playing music at 4 a.m. and being a general nuisance.

MYTH:

My surroundings will sculpt me into a different person and change my habits overnight.

REALITY:

Getting a semi-cool job and a new flat was not going to make me automatically fall into step with the rest of the tote bag-wielding, flower market-attending, natural wine-drinking and small plate-eating modern London creatives. My habits didn't change overnight and neither did the way I felt inside.

Prior to starting at the Beeb, I had to endure a fairly rigorous background check. It may seem standard enough, but as somebody who had more gaps on his CV than a secretive businessman with the hint of a German accent in Buenos Aires in 1947, I was pretty nervous. All the references I had put down on my resumé were imaginary. I had never been involved in feature films. Nor had I attended university. There was no degree on the mantelpiece. There wasn't even a mantelpiece. My relevant work experience consisted of poetic licence interspersed with complete fiction. Fortunately, the woman conducting the checks turned out to be a massive Westlife fan and overlooked the flagrant discrepancies on my CV in exchange for tickets to a non-existing Westlife reunion gig that I promised would be happening within a few weeks of me starting the job. I'm so sorry, Barbara.

In any event, after spending six weeks or so going back and forth between Dublin and London, dining out on the fact that I had been offered a position in the BBC and partying from one end of the week to the other, it was time to get to work. I was fucking terrified. This was the part I hated. On paper I should have been more than confident; the role I was hired for involved creating social media campaigns for scripted comedy and essentially required a decent knowledge of TV and the ability to be funny on the internet – my bread and butter – but I was hyper aware of the fact that I had failed to disclose a vital piece of information about myself during the interview process – I liked to go drinking. You might even go as far as to say that sometimes I preferred drinking to working. I knew something would have to change if this was going to work out properly. My hand had been forced by circumstance and I had a real opportunity to change as a tiny trade-off for the career that I wanted. I had spoofed my way into the BBC without a college degree and there was no way I would let something as trivial as *a few pints* get in the way of my success. It was time to turn a corner and close the chapter on all of those years of problematic drinking and drug-taking. Up until this point, any declaration of transformation was only ever made red-eyed after a binge, when I was delicate between the ears and not operating at full capacity. This time, however, it would be different. I wanted a consistent course of direction in life and the BBC was pretty much as reputable an organisation as it got ... notwithstanding, of course ... well, you know ... but ...

I panic-bought two outfits from Uniqlo and a couple of V-neck jumpers from COS in an attempt to make myself resemble what I believed to be the picture of the functioning modern man. Rather than abstaining from cocaine midweek or going for pints on a Monday, I thought that a beige pair of chinos would be the missing link between me and a life of consistency; that would be the ticket! Perhaps if I ditched my usual uniform of a cigarette-burnt leather jacket and black skinny jeans, I would be more organisation-friendly and less likely to stick out like a sore thumb? I still stuck out like a sore thumb.

The nine-to-five life was completely alien to me and hit me like a punch in the face. It was more of a culture shock than a career change. After a decade on the peripheries I was out of the loop when it came to the dynamics of the office, with its own rules and dialogue. It turns out that free-styling my way through my twenties with songwriting, nightclub promoting, robot selling, gig running and general spoofing had occasionally paid me well, but had at no point provided me with the required glossary or cheat sheet to adapt comfortably to the corporate world. I was barely even house trained. I remember in my first week casually telling one of my colleagues to 'get fucked' as a joke, when she asked me to do something, and I nearly got sent to HR. My early days in the organisation were like when a plumber or handyman fixes something in your house and then explains to you how he did it. You nod along knowingly, grunting at appropriate intervals as if you have any understanding of what he's on about.

I still remember my first day on the morning commute. It was as if I'd fallen asleep at the age of 24 and woken up at 28 in the middle of the rat race. Where had all the time gone? Where had all of my life gone? Suddenly I found myself feeling old, caught in the depraved mundanity of nine-to-five life and the monotony of Pret a Manger, Microsoft Teams, Winter Wonderland, rooftop bars, Hinge Prompts, Barbour jackets, *The Great British Bake Off*, Sally Rooney, Columbia Road flower market, house plants, Chilly's water bottles, Veganuary, *Love Island*, ASOS deliveries, VEJA runners, Joe Wicks, trainers on the Tube, Kygo, fold-up bikes, ironic tote bags, small talk over cupcakes on colleagues' birthdays, couch to 5Ks, mini golf and team pizza, park runs, unfunny memes on Slack, circling back, touching base, hating to chase, tomato-stained lunchboxes, Casa Amor, brunch culture, World Cup syndicates, selfies on swan-shaped pool toys, Greggs vegan sausage rolls, fresh Sundays, food markets ... it was all a great big rush to somewhere that I knew I never wanted to be.

Initially, things started out well, just like they always did. I was creating social campaigns for some of the biggest TV shows in the UK, in the

nexus of British comedy, and making a name
for myself in the teams I worked with. As is
customary, I celebrated finishing my first day
in the office by going out and getting shitfaced.
The venue was Soho House on Dean Street and
I went with an old friend. I drank about 11 pints
of Stella Artois and snorted poppers until my
lips turned blue. Poppers had become the sort
of 'healthy alternative' I reached for whenever
I couldn't get my hands on cocaine, a bit like
substituting a wholemeal wrap in place of white
sliced pan when you're making yourself a ham
sandwich. For those of you unfamiliar, poppers,
or amyl nitrite, are a liquid drug that can give an
instant high when inhaled. They are typically
considered unsafe for people to take.

I recall the awkward moment when I suggested
to my friend that we should order some drugs. I
still remember his face. A mixture of confusion
and concern. Quite similar to when you put your
coat on but don't grab the lead to bring the dog.
The wounded look of horror that he gives you. As
if to say, 'What? *Why*? Why would you do this?' I
often laugh thinking about the faux-casualness
of asking somebody if they're up for getting
some coke. As if the thought had just crossed my

mind, almost like I was surprised by it, and not that I had been plotting it since the very moment we sat down at the table. The high-pitched, almost throwaway nature of asking was all part of the routine, you see. Like a child working up the confidence to ask his parents if he could go to a party in the house of a boy they deem a bad influence. I'd beat around the bush with banal conversation until eventually launching the question out there, with forced indifference, as if I wasn't even that bothered and it was merely a suggestion *for the table*. Like a bowl of onion rings or a bottle of sparkling water.

My friend had foolishly assumed that we were just having a couple of pints and a catch-up as it was a Tuesday, politely declining my offer of narcotics as he was planning on calling it after four. Ah yes, the elusive *four*. I had heard about those. In fact, I had been chasing those four pints since my very first days in Brighton when I was only 18. I didn't even want them, deep down. The *casual four* after work on a Thursday just to ease yourself into the weekend, before picking up a takeaway on the way home, maybe feeling a little bit groggy on Friday but still functional enough to carry out your duties in a responsible manner. The *chilled-out four.* What an utterly insane concept. How could somebody go out for four drinks and then say, 'Do you know what? That's me. I don't think I fancy another one. I'm going to go home now and watch a Netflix documentary about a missing child who kidnapped his own parents.' It still seems insane to me, so *normal,* the way some people drink. For many years, I tried to practise my way into drinking *normally.* But every time I found myself reaching the end of that fourth pint, there would always be a very valid reason for me to continue drinking long after. Here's a few examples of the type of excuses I would use when contemplating the fifth pint:

1. You haven't seen this friend in ages.
2. The weather is good.
3. Come on, Mark, your mental health has been so poor recently, isn't it great for the soul to be out and about and doing a bit of living? This is basically *therapy.*
4. If you wait around a bit longer you will almost certainly meet the woman of your dreams.
5. You've just opened another box of cigarettes.
6. Six pints is a healthy number of pints. Four pints is anti-social.

The novelty of working in the BBC wore off after about two weeks when I realised that television was just as mundane as any other industry I had previously flirted with working in. There was no escaping a Monday. The same old problems started to creep in. The work wasn't interesting enough, they expected too much of me, the organisation was out of touch, they weren't doing things the right way, they weren't paying me enough, I wanted to be doing a different job from the one they hired me for, they didn't understand what was funny, there was too much red tape, the entire organisation was crippled by bureaucracy, blah blah blah. *Same old, same old.* Here I was, finding myself again at a crossroads. I was 27, unhappy in my life and with no idea how to change it. Oh, and of course I was drinking. I started missing work, missing meetings, missing deadlines ... old habits refused to die. The new career hadn't resulted in the personal transformation that I had anticipated, and that devastated me.

It's such an uncomfortable realisation, arriving at another destination and learning that it's not where you wanted to be in the first place. Whether it's a relationship, a job, a house, a holiday or an expensive jacket, the level of anger you feel at yourself after investing your time, money and effort into convincing yourself (or others) that this thing is *the* thing that will make you happy, only to discover that it's not, is a tough pill to swallow. Not only that, but now that you've gone ahead and taken the wrong turn, you also have to deal with two additional challenges: first, you have to accept defeat and admit that it was the wrong road to take, which is a lot easier said than done; and second, you have to figure out how to get back to the place you once were and to decide where to go from there. I burst into tears one night in a pub with a friend, thinking about how unfulfilled I was and how lost I felt in life. I was immediately so overcome with embarrassment at my sobbing that I quickly made up a lie about having personal issues with a family member in order to justify the tears, because I was too ashamed to tell him the real reason – that I had finally got the life I thought I wanted but all I wanted to do was drink. This emotional offloading with zero follow-up action quickly became my party piece. Some people do that annoying thing with their foot raised in the air to make it look like they're levitating, others lose phones or bank cards on nights out; I'd well up and talk about the death of optimism while doing absolutely nothing to change my circumstances the morning after. Eight pints on a Tuesday, telling a friend that I needed a new career and to curb my drinking while deliberating over whether or not to order a bag was my version of *the diet starts tomorrow.*

I rejected the nine-to-five culture thereafter because I failed at being a part of it. My antics and gallivanting on nights out rendered me incapable of doing anything other than isolating during comedowns and made it impossible to nurture steady relationships that weren't dependent on alcohol or drug-taking. I was dating a lot at the time but with little consideration for the other people involved. As far as I was concerned, dates were just another vehicle for getting bananas drunk, skating across the surface level of conversation and temporarily escaping the realities of life. Anything after that was a bonus. For a while, I thought of myself as quite the Lothario, to be honest, living spontaneously in the big city and leaving a trail of broken hearts behind me. There was definitely a trail of something. I thought I was a real heartbreaker for not texting girls after first dates, a desirable cartoon villain who was too bloody busy for matters of the heart. Then one day a woman rang me after we'd been on a date together the day before (11 pints, Sunday afternoon, work the next morning, etc.). I woke up to about three missed calls from her that Monday, and after sending screenshots of the missed calls to my best mate and commenting on how 'mental' she must have been, I eventually relented and rang her back. Preparing myself to make a grandiose speech about not being tied down to one woman and how comedians are designed to be alone, etc., my thoughts were interrupted when she blurted out straight away, 'Are you okay, Mark?' I was lost for words. 'Eh, what?' She continued, 'Listen, it doesn't matter if we see each other again and I know that we don't know each other, but I just wanted to check if you were okay and if there's anything you need to talk about? I can be here for you as a friend.' I acted like she was crazy, laughed at her and then proceeded to drunk text her for about six weeks at around 2 a.m. looking to link up. But deep down, something struck a chord. Beneath the ceaseless noise of my entertaining nonsense, she heard a plea for help. I wasn't quite as good at appearing normal as I thought I was.

Another time, I went to Battersea Park in the middle of a heatwave and drank five bottles of rosé with a girl from Newcastle before literally running away from her into the shrubbery like a seasoned loon without any reason or explanation. I genuinely wasn't even aware of how the evening ended until the next day when she texted me, 'Where did you run off to?' In my naivety, I assumed that was just a colloquial Northern mating call, or a hungover attempt at flirting, but after speaking to her on the phone it transpired that I had literally stood up in the middle of a conversation, delirious drunk, and shouted something insane, before sprinting off into the night towards Battersea Bridge.

You might wonder how I maintained this lifestyle financially. The simple answer is that I didn't, really. Every penny I earned went towards drinking, cigarettes, fast food and cocaine, so I could never afford things like a holiday or a new pair of shoes. If I wanted to go to the dentist, I'd have to phone home. When things got bad, I borrowed from my friends. Once or twice I availed of the insidious 'help' of a payday loan company, which I never told anybody about, and it took me almost two years to clear those debts. Haircuts were a luxury. At times

I walked to work because I didn't have enough money in my bank account to tap on for the Tube. If there was a demand for DVDs, you better believe I would have sold them all. Every time my money ran out, I'd swear it would be the last time. I would live like a pauper for a couple of weeks, eating pasta with one-pound sauce, promising I'd make a change, knowing that this was a tough but valuable lesson to learn when it came to drinking and doing drugs. Then payday would arrive with all its temporary euphoria and my money would go straight back up my nose and behind a bar. I was the definition of a weekend warrior. I definitely gave off the impression to people that things were a lot different financially from how they really were.

I'm sure it was obvious to some of those looking on – the ones afforded with objectivity, not close enough to be part of the circus or privy to my never-ending, contorting excuses and deceptive rationale, but the ones just on the outside, who could see me for what I really was, that something wasn't right. I remember showing up to a work-organised pizza and beer party one evening – which consisted of people mostly eating pizza (strangely enough), and the very odd person nursing a bottle of beer. I was visibly hammered and immediately looked out of place. I will never forget the look in people's eyes, mostly of concern rather than judgement. They were soft and worried and perhaps even a little afraid due to my unpredictable mood, but they were understanding. And they were a kind bunch, my colleagues. It's a shame that I didn't work harder at building better relationships with them. They were interesting, layered, kind, complex and passionate people with whom I shared many similarities. We were pretty much all nerds in our respective fields and thus enjoyed the contagious enthusiasm of being around other people doing work they adore. Eventually, though, I would only allow myself to see the differences. It was easier that way.

I stopped sitting near the wider team pretty soon after joining, because that meant I was able to slip off a bit earlier in the evenings and nobody would have to sit close to me and get the smell if I had been out on the pints the night before. Some people are very lucky when they drink; the booze doesn't get into their glands and under their skin. With me it was always porous. The fumes would seep out of me throughout the day like the leaky carcass of a beached whale. That unmistakably familiar scent of morning-after liquor would hover, with a layer of light and sticky sweat covering my skin, adding to my problematic glow. I tried to hide it. My routine when walking into NBH (National Broadcasting House) in the mornings would be to smoke at least five cigarettes, stop in the Boots near Bond Street Tube station and spray myself down with the sample bottle of L'Homme by Yves Saint Laurent, drink a strong coffee from Pret and then double-check that I was armed with enough menthol- and floral-scented products to see me through the day; miniature Listerine, Airwaves chewing gum, peach deodorant, coconut moisturiser, white Tic Tacs … The contents of my tote bag resembled that of a teenage girl's purse on the way to her first disco. I don't go rooting through teenage girls' purses, by the way. That's an observation from memory rather than a recent fact-find. I haven't been out scouring the cloakrooms in local community halls or GAA clubs in an attempt to prove this theory. I'm probably wrong anyway. Teenage girls' purses these days probably contain vapes, energy drinks and more cocaine than I brought across the Irish Sea from Holyhead. I don't know. We should probably stop talking about teenage girls' purses now, anyway.

As my disenchantment with life in the BBC grew, so did my drinking. I never drank on the job (unless I was working remotely, which was twice a week, so yes, I drank on the job) but I would often struggle to see through a full day in the office due to the lingering effects of the night before. There were a couple of close calls but mostly I seemed to get away with it. Or perhaps British people are just more polite than Irish people and wouldn't come out with something direct like, 'Hey, man, quick one, how many pints did you have last night? Because you smell like literal death.' One time, I was having a catch-up with a senior colleague in Television Centre in White City about an upcoming campaign I was working on. We were sitting in a little glass booth in the hot desk area. As we sat down, I reached into my jacket pocket to get some chewing gum, lest the smell of booze make the short one-foot journey from my throat into her nostrils. As luck would have it, the bracelet that I was wearing at the time got snagged on the stitching of my pocket. I pulled my hand aggressively and repeatedly, until the bracelet broke free and the chewing gum came flying out, along with a little rectangular betting slip packed full of cocaine. It then lay on the floor between us, unacknowledged. (For the uninitiated, some drug dealers wouldn't deliver the goods in plastic baggies, opting for a folded-up old betting slip instead. I had wasted hours looking for that bag the previous weekend, only to assume that it had been lost to the night.) I then spent the next five minutes sweating, completely unable to process a single world of what my colleague was saying, while the betting slip stayed on the ground, equidistant between us. Every now and then her eyes would wander towards the floor and I would bark or grunt or howl or squeal or do something equally weird in an effort to disrupt her line of thinking and to force her into focusing on something else. That was one of the closest calls I had ever had and I remember promising myself not to be that reckless again, while inhaling the remnants of the betting slip in the pub that evening, next door to the office. To this day I don't know if she saw the paper slip.

Another morning, I got an email from my line manager's line manager asking me to come into NBH for a physical meeting. The formality of a sit-down meeting came as a bit of a surprise and

it arrived on the back of me spending six consecu-
tive days *working from home*, so I knew that something was probably awry. In reality, the few days
working at home had been a week-long bender,
because I'd just started seeing a Turkish woman
twice my age who happened to enjoy drinking
to the same extent as me. She didn't work, so she
was always up for getting pissed during the day.
We would wander around central London, going
to the theatre, sniffing poppers and drinking our
way through the establishments of Soho while
I'd send the occasional email from my phone just
to keep up appearances. I would stay in her house
most nights, and in the mornings she'd send me
off to work with a pocket full of lunch money
and freshly washed socks. Until the dreaded but
predictable moment came when she got tired
of all of the drinking and confronted me about
it, suggesting that maybe we just *slow down* and
take it easy and do all the things I hated to do, like
going for walks or getting to know each other
properly. Next to 'not tonight' or 'your drinking',
I think 'slow down' was the last thing I ever
wanted to hear somebody say. You see, asking me
to slow down is like asking an Oklahoma garden
chair to dictate the course of its direction when

swallowed up by a tornado. The luxury of choice is no longer on the table once I have had a drink.

Back to the line manager's line manager. I had been summoned and I was terrified. The BBC usually adhered to a strict and glacial policy when it came to getting anything done, so for me to be called in on a whim definitely spelled danger. I retraced my steps from the week before and wondered who might have seen me. Perhaps it was a boring old office worker from a different department and they'd recognised me outside a bar in Soho, drunk at 3 p.m., and reported me to my team? Maybe somebody had slipped out to go to the dentist and had seen me in Soho House, Greek Street, laptop shut and bleary-eyed at lunchtime, guzzling a pint of Stella? Either way, I knew I was done for. I made my way to the Tube, the smell of booze still oozing out of me. Nothing would get rid of it. I practically basted myself in Jo Malone like a Thanksgiving turkey or a South Dublin mum doing the school run, but I couldn't shake it. All of a sudden the God that I used to sneer at people for believing in seemed like a fairly attractive entity to call upon for help. Making my way out of the station at Oxford Circus, I was metaphorically down on my knees: 'Heya, big man, listen, I know it's been a while since we last spoke. Well, specifically, in 2018 when I was on a flight to Barcelona and I thought the plane was going to crash ... But yes, it's me again and I need your help. I've really done it this time. I'm about to lose my job and I don't know what to do. If you help me out just once, I promise I will do anything you want. I will never drink again. That much is *certain*. I've learned my lesson. This is no way to live and I will be for ever in your debt if you could just save me my job.'

I walked through the doors of the BBC, trying to avoid eye contact with the security guards lest they rugby tackle me on the spot and search my person for more misplaced betting slips, and quietly entered the meeting room, sheepishly and sweaty. I offered my line manager and my line manager's line manager a brief, pleading smile, as if to say 'Please don't make me redundant' in the most David Brent level of *pity-me* poignancy I could muster up. They paused for a moment before asking me how my morning was. I told them it was fine. They then proceeded to inform me that my current role and the role superior to mine were being dissolved and that they would like me to step up and interview for a new position that would encompass both roles, with a salary increase and additional responsibility, as they'd be merging the two into one. Essentially, I was being offered a promotion. *Let's fucking go.*

I left the meeting room and walked straight around the corner into a bar on Great Portland Street to get a pint and settle my nerves. Between the shakes and the adrenaline, I didn't know my arse from my elbow. The one thing I knew for certain was that I was a very, very lucky boy. I spent the next few days on a binge to end all binges and made absolutely no changes to my lifestyle thereafter. Sure, why would I? I was blowing all of my worries out of proportion before, I couldn't be doing that badly if they're offering me a promotion, could I? My unorthodox work ethic was clearly working extremely well, and if anything, the promotion was proof. It was often an attractive notion to buy into the idea that maybe I just had an anxiety problem rather than a drinking problem.

This way of living would go on for months. Wednesday–Sunday were my drinking days. I would try to keep a lid on the Wednesday nights with just a few pints, but by Thursday all bets were off. Working from home on Fridays meant that I didn't even need to be upright on those mornings, so all I had to do was to keep my diary clear of one-on-one meetings and I would be able to lie in bed all day, slowly coming back to life, while absent-mindedly clicking the mouse to make it look like I was online, celebrating the upcoming weekend with a can of Red Stripe. Each week it was the exact same; I would start off my Monday in the depths of despair, riddled with so much remorse and self-loathing that I would often be incapable of even opening an email, only for the clouds to slightly part by Wednesday, offering a glimmer of hope and enough light to lend me the confidence to cautiously pick up a drink again, for that very drink to cause a chain reaction which would result in a four- or five-night binge until I would eventually run out of steam at some point on Sunday, falling into bed, exhausted, only to stare at the ceiling sleeplessly for six hours, dizzy with the anxiety and unspeakable intrusive thoughts, before wearily crawling out of bed on a Monday morning and starting the whole process all over again. And on and on it went. The highs got lower and the lows kept me wanting to get high. I was trapped.

CHAPTER 7

GOING DRY, WONDERING WHY

started trying to get sober in the autumn of 2019. There had been several attempts over the previous few years, many shaky mornings and sleepless nights devoted to swearing off the stuff for life, only for the conviction to all but dissolve by the time the weekend came around. I was sick of the Monday morning routine, voice noting my best friend Stuart, frantically pleading with him for reassurance that everything would be okay if I just committed to getting dry. Another year had gone by and it was as if my foot was caught in the spokes of a hamster wheel and I was slowly rotating my way towards insanity. I would like to say the previous 12 months had been action-packed with wall-to-wall madness, throwing television sets out of hotel windows, banging lines with celebrities, that sort of thing – and of course there had been a little bit of that – but for the most part, life had become very dull. Each week was a mirror to the last. Cocaine provided me with a sense of momentum and the illusion that things were happening, but the reality was that I was spending most of my free time sitting around kitchen tables in strangers' flats, wide-eyed and vacant, half having conversations over the passing of a kitchen plate and demanding an audience for obscure songs that I had found on YouTube. My mental health was deteriorating too, quicker than the Bulgarian timeshare market in the summer of 2009, but of course I couldn't bring myself to ask for help. It felt like I was looking out of the window of a moving train, watching the lives of my friends and family go by as they reached new milestones, celebrated achievements, processed bereavements and generally matured with age, while I was caught in the bear trap of non-stop drinking. Shamefully, when news of promotions, marriages, mortgages or marathons reached my ears, it was only ever met with envy. The resentment I held for my own circumstances interfered with my ability to be happy for those around me. I was miserable.

Ultimately, I made the decision to give it all up when I went back to Dublin for a wedding and got arrested the night before the ceremony. Well, nearly arrested. In the end, I think I only received a formal caution. From what I remember, I got into an argument with a taxi driver on the dual carriageway about 15 minutes from my father's house, after convincing myself that the driver was tampering with the meter in order to charge me an extra euro or so for the journey. (You'd think if somebody had the technological skills or desired computer wizardry to hack into their own taxi meter, they would probably adjust the fare to reflect a figure slightly larger than the price of a Freddo bar, but no, *not me*.) We argued for about 20 minutes until he became exasperated and decided to call the police. As luck would have it, the nearest Garda station was only 90 seconds from where the taxi stopped, so the police arrived on the scene about an hour later. I was quite belligerent and flatly refused to pay for the fare, which resulted in an altercation with the garda followed by an ill-timed visit to the family home by squad car.

I'm pretty sure that I even opted for the infuriating 'I know my rights' approach, which as we
all know is only ever used by people who do not
know their rights. It's a statement deployed by
phone-wielding neanderthals who feel the need
to record every encounter they have with the Irish
police because they've spent too much time on
YouTube and conflated the complex societal woes
and systemic racism of America with their own
inability to follow government restrictions during
a global pandemic. On the night in question, I was
drinking whiskey and subsequently blamed that,
the *uisce beatha*, for my aggression. One thing is
for certain, though, my head was in a strange
place. Earlier that evening, I had received a text
from my new housemate back in London (I had
moved flats again, around the corner in Fulham)
asking if I was okay. I replied in the affirmative
and questioned why he was asking. He told me
that the night before I left, he had found me face-
down on the couch, barely conscious and beginning to choke on my own vomit. I had come back
from the pub very drunk with my usual corner
shop haul – two packs of Pall Mall and a couple of
bottles of Casillero del Diablo – and apparently he
had to lift me up, get me to my feet and whack me

hard on the back so that I could clear the airways and continue to regurgitate the contents of a 10-hour binge, while putting me in the recovery position. I remembered none of it.

After the wedding, I went back to London feeling bruised and with my tail between my legs. Usually, I would crisis-call my therapist at times like this, when the lows got particularly low, demanding that she provide me with an insulin shot of emotional support to see me through the comedown, before casually disregarding the contents of the conversation once the wounds scabbed over and the itch to go out presented itself again. I did nothing to address my permanent 'all or nothing' thinking styles, so these eleventh-hour therapy sessions were totally redundant. It was all just papering over the cracks and a lazy, last-ditch attempt at avoiding the darkest of thoughts. Because they did get really dark at times. I came close to phoning the Samaritans once or twice, but my embarrassment got in the way and I convinced myself that I wasn't bad enough *yet* to warrant their time and that I shouldn't be clogging up the phone lines. It wasn't like that this time around. This time, I sat into the sadness instead of distancing myself from it and made no attempt to hide from the shame I felt.

I knew then that the only way out of this perennial loop of self-destruction was complete sobriety. The intervention I had been expecting might never arrive.

I had become very good at disguising the *bad*. There were always two separate trains of thought operating at any given time. The first was whatever I was experiencing in that moment and the second was the countless issues that required addressing and problems that needed to be solved – a conveyor belt of unpaid bills, unexplained absences from work and the general drama that came with dating people as insane as myself. I do know that I was particularly stressed that weekend as I had recently humiliated myself in front of a very senior and extremely sober colleague at a work party. I'd also had to move into yet another new flat after my landlord had given me my notice. In addition there was the *palme d'or* of wankery – my membership of Soho House had been suspended due to a fight I couldn't remember that I'd got into with a member of staff. I then got into a messy row with my brother on the weekend of the wedding. Finally, I'd lost the most treasured item I owned

– a bracelet given to me by my mother – after letting a stranger try it on when I was drunk. The list goes on and on, innumerable mundane and completely avoidable problems that came with the territory of my drinking. One thing was clear, the gaps between the dramas created by my binges were decreasing. Yet still, somehow, the word 'alcoholic' was not something I came close to uttering. At this stage I just had to stop drinking entirely because I wasn't in a great place. Bafflingly, the penny still didn't drop that I 'wasn't in a great place' because of my drinking.

Lots of memories from that period are hard to recall, not just emotionally but literally – most of the months just melt together into a formless blur, uncharacterised by the usual governance of time. Recollections from nights out were increasing in their scarcity too and I started to experience blackouts. Growing up, I thought that a blackout was when you lost consciousness or collapsed on your feet, but I had no idea of what it actually entailed. According to Google, 'alcohol-related blackouts are gaps in a person's memory for events that occur while they are intoxicated. These gaps happen when a person drinks enough alcohol to temporarily block the transfer of memories from short-term to long-term storage – known as memory consolidation – in a brain area called the hippo-campus. The most common type is called a "fragmentary blackout" and is characterised by spotty memories of events, with "islands" of memories separated by missing periods of time in between'. That little three-sentence biography summed up my drinking perfectly, and the persistent memory lapses of those years have definitely taken their toll.

Back in Fulham, I spent a week on my knees, picking up the pieces, writing out diet plans and deciding what marathons to run. I was now a non-drinker and I knew that winning Ironman races and becoming employee of the month in the BBC was the only plausible exchange for this monastic way of life. I started following all of the sober living Instagram accounts, penning the announcement for when I'd been six months off the stuff and doing lots of research on One Year No Beer and other forms of teetotalism. After seven days of abstinence and one sober Bumble date, I plucked up the courage to do something else that I had been threatening to do for a long time – I listened to a supportive friend, Neil, instead of the innumerable inner critics, and I started a podcast.

I had met Neil for a drink in Dublin the weekend before and he had reminded me of the ever-growing world of podcasts, trying to convince me that it would be a good vehicle for my style of comedy. I told him that I wouldn't even know where to start and shamefully couldn't even afford the podcast equipment he had sent me the Amazon links to. By the time I got back to London, the recording gear was waiting for me, accompanied by a note with a simple message: 'Press record.' I deliberated over ideas and concepts for a few hours but very quickly landed on *The Sunday Roast* as a title and format. The next day I pressed record and on 4 November the first episode of the show was recorded in one take. Now, you'll have to forgive me for a second as I say something that is probably vomit-, stroke- and diarrhoea-inducingly earnest, but when *The Sunday Roast* was born, it felt like I was reborn. (I know!) It had been four years since I had put out any form of comedy and the podcast did a lot of good when it came to filling the void that I felt within. I was very lucky with it, too; the first episode amassed thousands of listeners within the first day and flew right to the top of the charts. Artistically speaking, it was as if I had returned from total obscurity and repositioned myself on the map of Irish comedy overnight. I was back.

* * *

Thirteen days later I started drinking again. Because that's what I do. And it was fine at first, just like it always was. This time I was sticking to only a few beers, anyway. A *casual four*. Beer never did anybody that much harm, did it? Maybe I'd have the occasional glass of wine, too, but that would be it. Beer and wine. That seemed like a responsible, almost French and, dare I say it, *sophisticated* way of reframing my relationship with booze. This time it would be different, I was sure of it. I deleted all the drug dealers' numbers from my phone (except for one, just for emergencies) and thought that if I only drank certain drinks, went to specific places and socialised with a select few people then I would be able to drink normally. I was now in a good place. I was happy. The podcast had brought about a connection to people that I

never knew I needed. I was developing a relationship with the listeners, an audience of Irish
people across the world, and it gave me a sense
of purpose, a powerful feeling of belonging; and
something else that I had been seeking since
first boarding the plane to Brighton – direction.
I had somewhere to go and somewhere to be.
Sundays became my favourite day of the week
– the least likely and most remarkable of turn-
arounds. I actually looked forward to the end
of each weekend, sitting down at the kitchen
table, poring over my notes from the previous
seven days and recording the show.

Alas, within a couple of weeks of the new
measured approach to alcohol, I quickly stopped
marshalling my intake and began using cocaine
again too. *Life is too short*, I said to myself. *If I can't
enjoy the success and the fruits of my own labour, then
what's the point in all of it anyway?*

MYTH:

All I need in order to stop drinking is willpower. If
the problem is created by myself then it can be
solved by myself.

REALITY:

Time has taught me that in order to experience a true transformation in life, it all comes down to doing everything *differently* rather than redoing the same things harder or better. I wish I knew that back then. I was still under the impression it was on me to figure it out. Even when wanting to do the right thing, I was still desperately trying to control all of the outcomes. I wanted to be in the driving seat because that is where I felt the safest. Yet in reality, that's where I was in the most danger.

It was around then that I discovered Monday night drinking, and at first I thought I was a genius, I honestly felt like a fucking scientist. Drinking a little bit in the first half of the week countered the post-weekend blues and solved the crisis of the comedown. By *tapering*, I didn't need to crash-land into the working week with the grace of a spread-eagled pervert at your local swimming spot, hoping somebody will glance towards his genitals. A £4 bottle of Merlot from Sainsbury's in Fulham Broadway became the perfect antidote to the insomnia and night terrors that Mondays and Tuesdays usually brought.

There was a month or two when I was able to surf the waves of daily inebriation and spin the plates of life somewhat harmoniously. But what goes up must come down. As the success of the podcast grew, I became less interested in my work at the BBC and started to feel a gravitational pull to move back to Ireland. I was growing tired of London – *tired of life* – and I wanted to be in Dublin, surrounded by my family and taking advantage of the opportunity to do comedy full time that *The Sunday Roast* had afforded me. After a few months, the podcast was bringing in more per month than my BBC salary did, and some brands had started taking an interest in sponsorship too. Everything was going in the right direction. Well, actually, almost everything. The drinking and drug-taking had unfortunately kicked things up a notch too since *The Sunday Roast* started and the pendulum swings between wanting to stop drinking and then trying to drink like a normal person became more extreme, slowly depleting me of the ability to be happy.

I remember making my way home one night after a long day in the office – reeling from another sucker punch of a comedown – and standing on the crowded platform at Oxford Circus. Just as the train approached the station, the thought fleetingly crossed my mind as to what would happen if I stepped out in front of it. It wasn't more than a temporary urge but I considered it for long enough that my upper lip started to sweat and my heart began to race. In the end, I just got on the carriage, shaky and embarrassed, trying to distract myself from what had just happened by reading celebrity news on a stranger's iPad over their shoulder. It was time to go home.

I moved back to Dublin at the end of February 2020 and by the middle of March ... Well, we all know what happened then. Initially, I greeted the arrival of the global pandemic with the embrace of a grief-stricken mother cradling a wounded son returning from war. I relished the idea of life slowing down and grinding to a halt, just enough to get my bearings so I could gather my thoughts and really give things a proper go. I would finally get my shit together!

I didn't, in the end. While others baked banana bread and made dumbbells out of encyclopaedias, I reached for the old reliable and drank myself into oblivion at the kitchen table of my mother's house after she'd gone to bed, snorting poppers during Zoom quizzes and squandering all my Tinder likes. When the world stopped, I stopped. The podcast rambled on somewhat but failed to bring my spirit with it. Lockdown left me devoid of the stimulation that I didn't even know I required. I was done for, like a shark that stops swimming; without the framework of a regular life to at least somewhat subscribe to, I was governed only by instinct – and my instinct is to drink. I papered over the cracks with the odd sea swim and 5K run from Dún Laoghaire pier, but deep down, I knew I was slipping. I started hiding the drinking now too; occasionally bringing bottles upstairs and leaving them in the back of a sock drawer, quickly opening a new beer after hearing the sound of a car coming in the front gates just to make it look like I'd only started or meticulously placing the empties in the bottom of the bin underneath the other rubbish in the hope that they wouldn't get spotted. These little gestures of dishonesty formed a pattern of concealment that would only get worse with time. Cheap tricks that succeeded in their deception, but with the overall sleight of hand of a jaded magician doing the graveyard shift on a commercial cruise liner, the illusions did little to mask the general despair.

After some time and during a lull in the pandemic, I moved into a flat in Monkstown with two girls, Suzanne and Keeva, who were friends of friends, which heralded a new period of fresh starts and broken promises. *On the drink, off the drink, on the drink, off the drink.* A near-constant punching match between old habits and new beginnings. I would always have an excuse for either, depending on the mood I was in. Truthfully, I'm still haunted by the dichotomy between the mornings spent running 5Ks at sunrise and the shame of standing in my bedroom less than one day later with my ear to the door, waiting to hear the sound of the TV switch on in the living room before wrapping empty wine bottles in bath towels and stuffing them into a gym bag, just to sneak them out of the house without anybody hearing the clinking. How quickly the wind could change. I wanted to get sober but couldn't seem to figure out how. I started to think that perhaps I was a lost cause, completely insane and destined for asylum life, such was the frequency of the changes of heart I had when it came to alcohol and drugs. Some days I could be standing in the shower with a smile on my face, thinking about how happy I was to be clean, to be *free*, and that I never had to drink again, only to pick up my phone the moment I got back to the bedroom and to fire out WhatsApps to my friends to see if anyone was about that evening, along with the cursory 'Are you around?' message to my most reliable dealer – just as a precaution, so I wouldn't be left on the back foot or have to go without. Sometimes, I would even leave it in the hands of the gods – making promises and deals with myself, like 'Okay, well, you've texted the dealer now. If he doesn't get back to you in 15 minutes, then you have to take that as a sign and not go out tonight.' Sixteen minutes would go by and I'd pretend to read the clock wrong and send him the dreaded second text: 'Hey, mate, sorry for annoying you but just wondering if you'll be about soon because we're heading off from here in around half an hour.'

Covid also made it an awful lot easier and more socially acceptable to do cocaine at home. Or at least, during Covid *I* found it an awful lot easier and more socially acceptable to do cocaine at home. Due to the capricious nature of the travel restrictions, I tended to only meet up with one or two people at any given time, which was actually ideal for the type of user I was. If truth be told, I would have preferred to have been totally alone, but getting involved with another person gave me the sense that I was engaging in an activity – like climbing the Sugar Loaf or going to a spin class – and it helped delay the nagging 'what the fuck are you doing, it's a Tuesday' thoughts that would invariably set in, usually starting at the back of the head on snorting the first line, and arriving right between the eyes at around 7.48 a.m. The regret would reach a crescendo when the person I was with would utter the seven most appalling words that one can ever hear at a session, 'I think I'm going to call it', and suddenly I'd find myself outside their house, scrambling to find a cigarette while waiting for a taxi in the unforgiving glare of daylight, ears burning with birdsong and the other siren sounds of the working week. Even now, I struggle with the noise of birds chirping in the mornings. It's too vivid and it transports me straight back to those early mornings spent staring out of taxi windows on the way home from all-nighters, watching normal people go about their lives, wearing gym gear or walking dogs, ready for the world. I hated them and was jealous of them all equally. My destructive drinking was severing the lines of connection to other people, making it even less attractive to stop. I believed I was fundamentally different from the average person and unable to get along with life, making it a lot easier to justify those three-day benders. I didn't realise how easily I would be able to 'get along' when not blowing up my life each weekend with intense, 15-hour sessions of heavy drinking and drug use.

Gradually, as certain as death, taxes or an American tourist getting over-excited in a teppan-yaki restaurant, my work began to suffer too and the podcast started slipping, in both relevance and regularity. Recording inconsistencies meant a dip in the quality, as weeks would go by where I'd be lost to the session and devoured by its aftermath, only to come back in a flurry one random Sunday afternoon, flooding the airwaves with promises, guaranteeing a regime change and breaking the news of a new sheriff in town, before time would reveal that this new sheriff was, in fact, also an alcoholic. I was somehow just about holding on to my job in the BBC via remote working, but I was still availing of copious mental health mornings and sick days; it wasn't going to last much longer.

I was reckless. One afternoon I went to the park with a friend and decided that I would only drink the one bottle of wine and do a *baby* bump, because I had a team meeting at 3.30. Sense had leapt out of the window. Again, I probably have British politeness to thank for keeping me in the job that day because any human on that Zoom call with a working frontal lobe would have noticed that I was definitely drunk. In December 2020, I left the BBC to pursue comedy full time. Looking back, I was fortunate enough to be able to walk out the door while it was still a choice. I wonder what would happen if I ever tried to walk back through those doors.

At some point during the aeons of Covid-19, I got into a new relationship. It felt like the right thing to do at the time, and perhaps the partying was just a result of being single – maybe if I had someone to watch movies and climb mountains with, I wouldn't need to go out drinking as much? I can practically hear the sound of your eyebrows raising and face contorting into an *oh-for-fuck's-sake-Mark* expression as you read this. That's okay – mine would too. And, of course, you'd be right. It did absolutely nothing to ease the volume or frequency of my alcohol consumption, and in the end it unfolded and collapsed in the same way it began – with chaos. Lots of which can be attributed to my drinking. I foolishly thought that getting into a relationship would be a good reason to stop drinking when in reality it became the perfect excuse to continue.

Within a matter of weeks I was asked point blank if I had a problem. It felt like an accusation of gross proportions rather than a concerned enquiry about my wellbeing. Enter mock surprise from stage left, followed by the immediate recounting of how many drink-free days I'd had in the previous month and the observations of all the foolish things I'd seen the other person do when they were drunk, until eventually deploying the self-centred 'Do you not realise how much I've got going on?' and 'If only you knew how hard it is to be me maybe then you'd understand' emotional pleas as a grand finale. The well-oiled excuse machine was ready at all times to fire out a performance for any individual who dared question my penchant for ethanol. As long as I regaled enough stats in quick succession about how much I *wasn't* an alcoholic, I thought that would suffice.

With much reluctance and after several months of arguments, I agreed to see an addiction counsellor. I had already been to one therapist but I'm fairly sure that I managed to convince her that cocaine was the same thing as hash and that I only drank on Tuesdays. At this point, though, my behaviour was very erratic and visible to lots of other people – not just my girlfriend – and the 'partying' had become an impassable obstruction on the path to a stress-free existence. I'd also been caught out on a few occasions lying about what I'd drunk, who I was with, where I was, so it was clear that lots of things weren't how I said they were. At this stage, when I wasn't drinking, most of my time was spent dealing with the issues *caused* by my drinking. The whole thing was going pear-shaped and I was furious at myself for letting it get this bad. Truthfully though, I was even more angry at the person I was in a relationship with for highlighting the obvious truths and pointing out the behaviours that I had previously got away with.

Drinking several bottles of red wine until I was too drunk to finish recording a podcast was not normal behaviour. Doing drugs by myself at the desk in my bedroom while my girlfriend was asleep in bed is also not normal. Sneaking off into the bathroom to do baby bumps while she and my housemate were having a casual glass of wine and watching *Bake Off* on a Tuesday night is not the behaviour of a well-adjusted individual. Alas, resentment is one palatable drug. At times I felt that life had been a hell of a lot easier as a water-treading drunk in central London, with transient relationships – mostly drinking buddies – and spending my Sunday nights in soaking wet bedsheets, dripping with cold sweat rather than sitting in a flat in suburban Dublin at the other end of a pointed finger, being reminded of the terrible things I'd done the night before. I hated the fact that someone was seeing me for what I was. At least in London I was drowning on my own terms. You see, another addition to the limitless contradictions of this disease is that it was perfectly okay for *me* to harbour feelings of concern about my drinking and to express the desire to quit, but if somebody ever mentioned that I might indeed have a problem, all bets were off. Have you ever found yourself complaining to a friend about a family member? You want them to listen and to nod in agreement at the appropriate intervals, empathising with your frustrations, but should they decide to go rogue at any point and pass a comment themselves about your family member – well, that's cause for the instant dissolution of the friendship, as far as I'm concerned. It didn't make sense that I really wanted to get sober until I was told to get sober.

I approached my session with the addiction counsellor with delicate care, reaching deep into my wardrobe to dig out the old COS V-necks and a pair of beige chinos for the first encounter. I'm joking, of course. I was actually pretty honest with her – *to a point*. I was about as honest with her that day as I could be with myself – it was conditional, and only bits of the truth were drip-fed out. I was still manipulating, still deceiving and avoiding telling it exactly how it was. I crafted my story in a way that made me a lot more likeable and divulged enough of my own shortcomings to show her that I was being truthful, but held back on the gorier details when it came to how often I was drinking and taking cocaine. I focused instead on other issues like the unhappiness I felt in my relationship and how trapped I was, blaming the boredom of Covid for idle drinking, rather than my lifelong history of booze-fuelled escapism. After the first 30-minute session, the counsellor agreed that I was definitely drinking too much but that it might not yet require a life of total temperance. Yes! That was all I needed. I was not an alcoholic! *Thanks, doc!* Over 10 years on from that visit to the NHS doctor in Brighton and lo! I was still not an alcoholic! The pint-drinking passport had been stamped. I cherry-picked the most favourable things she said, made a few slight alterations and went home that evening with a grin glued to my face like an Essex bloke at a pool party who'd just bumped into Wayne Lineker. Pour me a cold one please, barkeep.

Within 72 hours, I was sitting in front of my GP with my head in my hands after a senseless binge. Red-eyed and sleep-deprived, I pleaded with him for the answers. That morning I had experienced the darkest thoughts possible and was worried for my wellbeing – but fortunately I had called my mother during a lapse in the fren-zied distress and had got myself up to the doctor's office. For the first time ever, I told somebody the full truth about my drinking. We explored all the options and he explained unequivocally that I needed to stop right now. (Thank you very much.) He gave it to me plain as day, in a series of logical, medical and fact-based statements. *You need to stop drinking, Mark. Before we even look at your physical health, it's clear that it's ruining your life.* I baulked when he mentioned the potential necessity for residential treatment and implored him to look at alternatives. We eventually agreed on a series of blood tests to see how the liver was doing and a commitment for me to engage in the other recovery options he had outlined. I was sent on my way with a prescription for Antabuse (yes, it's actually called that and is often pronounced 'anta-booze'). Antabuse is a daily tablet given to alcoholics to stop you drinking because if you drink when taking it, you get very sick, very quickly. A quick google about what would happen if I drank was enough to scare me straight and I knew that it wasn't an option. So I did what any normal person would do – I didn't fill out the prescription and instead went home to have a few beers. About eight bottles, just to help take the edge off. The *dry life* was going to take a lot of getting used to and I needed to ease myself into it.

From the next day, I was sober. It was late August 2021 and I had exhausted the patience of many of those around me with my various bouts of white-knuckled, ego-driven abstinence and this time it *had* to stick. I engaged in lots of surface-level self-help work, YouTube tutorials and motivational quotes, spoke to people I knew in recovery and stomped angrily around the house slamming doors and cursing everything. There's a video on the internet of the playwright John B. Keane describing a hiatus from booze and it's practically ASMR for someone like me. He poetically chronicles the agitation of short-term sobriety, beautifully capturing the unease and inner restlessness of being separated from life's greatest pacifier.

I think we both know that I had one drink left.

CHAPTER 8
LAST ORDERS

always thought my final drink would be a little bit different. In my head, there would be one last chance to say goodbye, perhaps an opportunity for some sentimentality, a melancholic adieu to my former friend, confidante, teacher, therapist and god. Maybe I would get a moment to be with it alone. I would ask why it turned on me and if there was anything I could do to change its mind. My head was clearly still rooted in fantasy as that wasn't to be the case at all. My last bender was just as confusingly plain as the rest of them. If anything, it was even less exciting, as it was really just an instinctive reaction to sobriety rather than a deliberate quest for drunkenness. Life without my usual anaesthetic was not something I was designed for and the six sober weeks leading up to the final binge were like swallowing cinnamon powder after a hike with no water. Everything was so fucking boring and I couldn't tolerate the idea of living like this permanently. Once the shame wore off and the usual amnesia kicked in after that visit to the doctor's office, I experienced the creeping suspicion that maybe everything had been blown out of proportion. I had tentatively looked into some recovery groups in my area but was hesitant to go any further than internet forums or self-help books about *drinking mindfully* because I automatically assumed that any place with chairs positioned in a semi-circle would be packed so densely with nutters that the room would probably resemble one of those overflowing Japanese commuter trains, bursting at the seams with loons.

I thus found myself caught in the stifling half-life of no longer consuming alcohol but not addressing why I drank in the first place either, resulting in a cripplingly strained version of sobriety that had my knuckles sheet-white and my emotions in a permanent state of disarray. I was in bits. After all, I *did* drink for a reason. At best, you could describe these weeks as tempestuous and I didn't really tell anybody that I was trying to stop for ever. It was easier that way. I spent a lot of time in my bedroom with the curtains drawn even in the middle of the day, trying to ration the amount of Instant Win Digital Cash Cards I played on the lottery website so that I wouldn't hit my daily allowance too early. It was grim. The addiction had to go somewhere, after all.

The gaps between the prison bars of active addiction were at least wide enough to give me glimpses of joy, whereas this type of sobriety, isolated and untreated, left me alone in a windowless cell, wallowing in the dark and observing my own slow demise.

Most of my friends and family were familiar with my on-again, off-again approach when it came to drinking, so very few questions were asked. As far as they were concerned, I was probably just a bit mad. I had always been inconsistent, after all. I approached new hobbies, friendships, jobs, etc. with intense enthusiasm at the very beginning, only to get bored after a week or two and start gravitating towards something else shiny and new. It's no surprise that my attempts at sobriety fell into the same category as 'exercise' or 'new creative projects'. They didn't see the days spent with the curtains closed or the sleepless nights of senseless rumination. Covid was still lurking in the shadows and it was more than acceptable to withdraw for a few weeks and to not make contact with those who you were close to. Throughout these withering stints of *dryness*, everything was quite numb and blurry – it felt like I had been neutered and was now a witness to life rather than a liver of it. The podcast had ground to a complete halt. I lost the energy to write a fresh script each week as I felt that I lacked the experiences required to provide inspiration. Comedy once again became a distant dream. My career had come to a bit of a standstill. The relationship I was in had also failed, but I was haphazardly trying to preserve it in an attempt to achieve some sense of control and order over my life. Alcohol may have caused lots of our problems but sobriety was not going to solve any of them. I was 30 years of age and it felt like the jig was up. The music had finally stopped.

I didn't plan on drinking at the wedding, it just worked out that way. Although I wasn't a willing participant on this newfangled journey of sobriety, I didn't intend on totally detaching myself from its meddling, interfering fingers just yet, either. I was prepared to endure a few more miles on the mundanity train and hopefully break my personal best of seven weeks without a drink – the longest I'd ever gone in adult life – before contemplating what the future might hold. My cousin was getting married right at the treacherous turning point of the six-week mark, so it was always going to be a challenge. The only time I'd ever gone longer without a drink was in 2020 when I had to get both of my wisdom teeth surgically removed before they became infected and I suffered from the unimaginable torture of a condition known far too inoffensively as *dry socket*. I wouldn't recommend it. Unless, of course, it was to be included on a tasting menu that contained other delights such as 'waking up during a colonoscopy when the sedation wears off' or 'the GP having to manually lift up your toenail before injecting a syringe straight into the soft part underneath'. In any event, I owed at least 18 days of those seven weeks of clean time to mind-numbing dental agony, when it would have been impossible to drink, even if I'd wanted to.

In advance of the big day, myself, my long-suffering girlfriend and another friend who was in recovery developed a series of getaway plans to help see me through the weekend. They contained Irish exits, emergency phone calls and rescue operations in the dead of night, should I need to vacate the place at short notice or if the desire to drink became too much. We covered every eventuality and left no stone unturned. I arrived at the hotel with my family the next day and I knew that I wasn't going to drink. I was in complete control. We drove out to the church and I knew that I wasn't going to drink. I was in complete control. We then made our way towards the location where the reception was being held and I looked at my phone. There were two messages on the screen. One was from my then girlfriend reassuring me that everything was going to be alright and to let her know if I was struggling, as she would drive across the country to collect me. The other was from my friend, who we will call F, wishing me well and reminding me that he was only at the other end of the phone should I need to chat at any stage. Nope, no thanks. It's too late. I ignore them both.

The phone goes on airplane mode and I decide to get drunk. When that happens, there is no point even talking to me. In fact, if you try, you are not only wasting your time, but you're really wasting my time. Any conversation that gets in the way of me drinking once I have decided to drink will be met with nothing but complete animosity. You're only slowing down the inevitable. I still remember that exact second in the car. It was as if my entire life had flashed before my eyes and I saw a vision of every single social situation, every birthday, every wedding, every bit of *life* that would happen in the future and I knew that the idea of doing it sober was far more depressing than any comedown from cocaine. I did not want to live in a world like that. There was a conversation going on between two family members in the front of the car about the various travel routes that one could take when driving back to Dublin the following day and the sheer force of how utterly incapable I was at being normal hit me in the face like the closed fist of a moron. *Of course* I was going to drink again. How could I not? I didn't feel like I had a choice, really. *Take me away from myself and out of this Godforsaken place*. The guilt was already forming a ball in the pit of my stomach but nothing was going to stop me now. *You can't put the toothpaste back in the tube.*

As soon as we arrived at the reception, I took a glass of champagne. Bang. Next. More champagne. My younger sister asked me if I was okay, as she thought that I had told her during the week that I wasn't going to be drinking that weekend. I was *grand*, I said, and sidestepped the inquisition. My head was screaming at me. I couldn't get the alcohol into me quick enough. It didn't seem to be working the way I thought it would, though. I wanted conviviality and ease. I was chasing a lightness that I once knew many years before, on teenage holidays and nights out with friends. I assumed that after the first drink my shoulders would sag joyously and my lungs would open up, breathing in the fresh air of life that surrounded me. The last few weeks had been so restrictive, both physically and mentally – I was wearing sobriety like a straitjacket – and I just wanted to be free like everybody else. It wasn't working. The internal noise was deafening and the voices inside my head were a constant chorus of '*What the fuck are you doing, Mark?*', I was walking around introducing myself to people, wondering why they had confused looks on their faces. 'Hi Mark, eh, we actually met just under an hour ago outside the church.'

Ah yes, but that was different. I wasn't *me* then. I was bored and despondent. I was sober, dry, dull and uninteresting. You name it. Now, though, everything has completely changed! Now I have my confidence back. There's colour in the world again. This was my terrain. I drank and drank until the last drop was poured in the residents' bar, crawled up to my room and collapsed on the floor of the bathroom in my clothes, only to wake up a few hours later, dizzy and dehydrated, but just about lucid enough to make out the vomit stains that covered the walls – you'd be forgiven for thinking it was a piece of bad art left over from the Celtic Tiger. I checked my phone. Endless, furious messages from the night before followed by one tiny, gentle, defeated text this morning. 'It's okay, Mark. Wherever you are, it will all be okay. Call me when you get up and we can get you back home. I love you.'

I turned my phone off and started drinking again. I couldn't face what awaited me in Dublin and took the only exit I knew off the road to reality. The day before had given me a taste for what I had been deprived of over the last few weeks – well, months really. All the stopping and starting had starved me of a proper, limitless bender and I was determined to chase that feeling, to trap it and to maintain the elusive buzz that had evaded me for so long. After a few settlers, I started trying to arrange the drugs. It was always easy to find other people who were interested in doing it but between the lack of phone coverage and the fact that we were somewhere in the back end of rural Carlow, it was quite the struggle to actually find a dealer willing to deliver. Eventually, I convinced my regular guy in Dublin to make the four-hour return trip with a couple of measly bags for the fee of €1,000. Rather fittingly, it would cost me practically every last cent I had in my bank account at the time. *May as well go down with a fight,* I thought. I needed something stronger as the booze wasn't cutting it. I don't recall much from the afternoon – once the drugs were on the way it was hard to think about anything else – but I continued drinking steadily while maniacally checking my phone every 30 seconds, hoping for an update on the delivery. If you're unfamiliar with this sensation, it's like waiting for the kettle to boil when you're dying for a cup of tea – you stand in the kitchen beside it, intensely willing time to move along quicker and urging the water to boil. Now imagine that feeling but with a kettle that produces cocaine and the cup of tea is a cup of cocaine.

In the early evening, a storm moved in and the day was swallowed by night. The dealer finally arrived and I wandered off in search of him on the grounds of the estate. Soon, after walking through the torrential rain, I was sitting in the front seat of his car, soaked through to the bone and with water dripping from my eyes. He kindly allowed me to snort a couple of bumps off the back of my phone before driving away and firmly reminding me that he'd need the money by Tuesday. I remember him glancing at me with a sort of 'You alright, mate?' look, just before I fell out of the car and stumbled back into the storm, heading towards the venue. Even my drug dealer had grown sick of the 'This is the last time, I swear' routine that I performed every time I saw him. It was done with as much conviction as a philandering douchebag in the locker room on a golf trip with the boys, distributing pictures of his latest sexual conquests while saying he shouldn't be cheating on the wife, all the time with a smile on his face.

On the way back to the party, I bumped

into my younger sister in the pouring rain and she immediately burst into tears. It turns out that my absence hadn't gone unnoticed and she had formed a little search party with one of my cousins to try and find me. My sudden disappearance had caused her to think the unthinkable and she was worried that I might have taken a turn and done something terrible. Perhaps I wasn't as good as I thought I was at convincing people I was doing okay? Usually when someone disappears from a wedding it's because they've got lucky and found their way into the arms of another individual who is experiencing the manic hunger for human connection that weddings can produce and they've ended up down a hallway somewhere, stuffing their tongues in each other's throats or doing intercourse standing up with their trousers down, cramped inside a broom closet. Suffice to say, that was not the case for me. I reassured my sister that everything was *fine*, and that I was *fine*, and we reintegrated with the other guests. I then stayed up until six or seven in the morning, working my way through the remainder of the bag and talking shite to whoever would listen, before eventually dragging myself to bed at sunrise when my body ran out of steam. I didn't get a wink of sleep. It was a dance as old as time.

At around nine o'clock in the morning, the dam burst, the levee broke and the tears arrived. Big, heavy, chest-heaving sobs that shook me from my skull to my feet. It was as if something in my brain had snapped and I just couldn't do it any more. I couldn't go on like this. I sat on the end of my bed and I cried like a little boy. For the first time in my life, I tasted true resignation. In the past, I may have met defeat but I had never known surrender. Alcohol had me every way it wanted me and I knew there was no escape. It felt like I was suffering from some sort of mental collapse – a dark night of the soul – and I spent 30 minutes bawling in front of my younger sister, labelling my relationship as the cause of all my pain but knowing deep down it wasn't the case. I had a much bigger problem. I *was* the problem. I was an alcoholic. It all descended on me at once in its huge, bewildering, devastating obviousness, while I sat on the end of that bed, blubbering like a baby, still in my clothes from the night before. Not long after, we had to leave. So I took the most Irish course of action I knew

– conjured up a smile, walked outside to meet the remaining wedding party, thanked the generous hosts for including me on their special day and went to load up the car. The ability to feign my own sanity clung on.

And that was it. I don't even remember my very last drink. It was probably a warm glass of white wine or a shared can of cider. The usual type of slop that would be left in the trough at six o'clock in the morning. Talk about an anti-climax. Fifteen years, several countries, new friends, old friends, lost friends, big highs, huge lows, late nights, long nights, and then it just stopped. And that was it. I always thought that my swan song would come with a press release. It would probably make the six o'clock news. At the very least, I expected it to include the flickering lights of police car sirens or a struggle with two orderlies as my flailing limbs got strapped to a steel gurney, en route to the madhouse. Instead, I sat in the back seat of my cousins' Hyundai on the drive back to Dublin, looking out of the window at the cars passing by and barely spoke a word, with a sore nose and a racing mind, contemplating the fact that life as I knew it was over. It was finished. We stopped in a McDonald's in one of the service stations off the motorway and I couldn't even eat my chips. *I* was finished. I was done.

The last day I took a drink or drug was 24 October 2021.

CHAPTER 9

THROUGH THE LOOKING GLASS

The week after the wedding, I sat down with my parents and gave them the unabridged version of my drinking. In the absence of knowing how to frame the story, I opted for the truth. My problems were now of a variety that transcended familial intervention, so there was little need to sculpt my predicament into anything more palatable. I was mentally, emotionally and spiritually fucked. They were tough conversations and I remember struggling to meet my father's eye. Truthfully, I was embarrassed. It felt like I was admitting to a crime of colossal proportions, born out of greed and stupidity rather than insecurity and fear. My parents had worked tirelessly for the previous four decades to provide the best life possible for my siblings and me, and it felt like a huge failing – a rejection of the life they'd afforded me – to have swerved the lanes of convention, insisting that I knew what I was doing while ignoring all the warning signs, only to crash-land onto their respective doorsteps at the age of 30, with tears in my eyes, admitting that I'd got it all wrong. I was worried that I would bring shame to my family by having a drinking problem – it wasn't exactly on the curriculum in St Michael's College and I don't recall anybody encouraging me to put it down on the CAO either. *And just what would the neighbours think?*

MYTH:

The consequences of telling the truth about my drinking would outweigh the suffering that my drinking induced.

REALITY:

I couldn't have been more wrong. Getting honest with my parents was the first step on the journey back to sanity. My aversion to vulnerability was so strong that I was more embarrassed about telling people that I needed help staying sober than I was about all the things I did when I was drunk.

The next step in the short term was admitting that I couldn't really trust myself when it came to staying sober for the long term, so I did the opposite of what my head was telling me and ditched the usual toolkit I reached for when trying to get off the sauce. This time there would be no visits to the GP's surgery, I wasn't going to call an addictions counsellor and I certainly wasn't going to grace the chaise longue of my ever-patient therapist, waxing lyrical about being misunderstood and saying that I only drank to cure my genius. That is not to undermine the value, effectiveness or potency of doctors or therapists – I have sought the help of both my GP and a counsellor at other intervals in my sobriety – but I just knew that I had to do things differently from before. I knew that I was an alcoholic. I didn't need to seek a medical diagnosis. I was spiritually sick, right to the core. The YouTube tutorials on healthy drinking went unwatched and the books on reframing bad patterns remained unread. I had conducted enough thorough research in the field to know the extent of my problems and that

I couldn't stop even when I wanted to. If left to my own devices I would certainly drink again – that much was a fact. My ability to stay sober without getting outside help was like the fable of the scorpion and the frog. In case you're unfamiliar, here's a brief synopsis, taken from the internet:

A scorpion wants to cross a river but it cannot swim, so it asks a frog to carry it across. The frog hesitates, afraid that the scorpion might sting it, but the scorpion promises not to, pointing out that it would drown if it killed the frog in the middle of the river. The frog considers this argument sensible and agrees to transport the scorpion. Midway across the river, the scorpion stings the frog anyway, dooming them both. The dying frog, with tears in its eyes, asks the scorpion why it stung despite knowing the consequence, to which the scorpion replies: 'I'm sorry, I couldn't resist. It's in my nature ...'

I am both the scorpion and the frog. Drinking is in my nature. If I were to repeat the same series of failed measures once more, it could result in dire consequences, of that I was certain. I was through the looking glass. There was no going back. This time I only made one phone call and that was to a friend who we'll call The Canadian, and I asked to be put in touch with a man he had spoken about before. He had a friend who had once known an appetite for cocaine and alcohol so voracious that it had almost destroyed his life, bringing him to his knees and nearly costing him his family and career. Remarkably, though, a few years ago there had been a dramatic turn-around and now he was completely clean, apparently living happily in the suburbs of Dublin with his family and totally free from the chaos and insanity of active addiction. From what I had heard about his drinking, he sounded *much* worse than me, so I felt like a conversation with him could be a good starting point. You might remember that I always found it beneficial to be around people who were worse than me. First when I was drinking and now when I was trying to stop. If a case more hopeless than mine could show signs of recovery, then it meant I stood a chance.

I picked up the phone, dialled the stranger's number – we'll call him *the most outrageous man,* sheepishly mumbled my way through the entire sob story – the same one I've just told you – and waited for his assessment. Halfway through, I realised that there was a chance he would tell me that I'd got it all wrong, that maybe I wasn't an alcoholic, and perhaps a life of abstinence wasn't going to be necessary. Maybe I should stop being so dramatic, just rein it in and lay off the bag? My voice cracked as I reached the crescendo of the most recent binge, raw with emotion and fragile inner defeat. It was met with total silence. Five seconds went by and still I heard nothing. *I knew I wasn't bad enough to be making a call like this, I was wasting the man's time. What the hell was I thinking in the first place? This was so embarrassing.* Finally, I heard a sharp intake of breath and braced myself for him to break the news that I was just a bit of a softie who probably liked the odd pint too much, when suddenly I heard the wheezy sound of giggling. The fucker was actually laughing at me. 'Oh yeah, you are completely fucked,' he said, and he burst out laughing. At that moment, I knew that I was on the phone to the right person. This was my kind of guy. *The most outrageous man.* A guy whose humour lived in the gallows, pulled no punches when it came to the mock derision of self or others, and best of all – he was sober! Almost instantly after the chuckles, his voice became more serious and he asked if I was truly ready to stop drinking and had I finished trying to do everything the Mark Mehigan way. I told him yes. He then recommended that I go and speak to other alcoholics. I said I wasn't sure what could be gained from chatting to a bunch of low-life drunkards, but he quickly reminded me that I too was a low-life drunkard. Fortunately, such was my desperation not to drink that I did exactly what he suggested and thus embarked on a journey unlike anything I had ever known.

Every night I would go and talk to other alcoholics. And every night I would begin to hate myself a little less.

The first few months of sobriety contained a profound simplicity that I often miss. Although it was a mournful time – I grieved the loss of alcohol as you might the loss of a limb – there was a quiet liberation that came with admitting to myself and others that I was totally *fucked*. Fifteen years of drinking had turned me into one tired little boy, and a huge amount of pressure had been relieved by throwing in the towel. I was still hopeless, of course, but at least now I had company. There *were* many others like me, it turned out. Countless men and women who also wanted to get sober and take things one day at a time. I found my tribe in groups of strangers who displayed the exact same irrational, unintelligible dependency as I did on a substance that was clearly fucking up their lives yet persisted in repeatedly trying to get a grip on its allure. Overnight, I became just one of many odd people rather than the odd one out. A black sheep in a flock of black sheep. After spending most of my life yearning to fit in, it took me finally giving up on everything to discover exactly where I belong. By opening up to people who didn't know anything about me, articulating my darkest thoughts about my urges to escape myself, the overwhelming feeling of *outsiderness* and my general inability to love myself, I was given a daily antidote to the manic thoughts of early sobriety, helping counter my instinctive tendency to withdraw from others and to isolate whenever I felt uncomfortable.

It wasn't going to be easy, though. I had become accustomed to the torrid limbo of resisting who I really was, languishing in a life of debatably functional alcoholism while keeping people at arm's length, so it was going to take a lot of work to break down the walls around me and dismantle the prison in which I had become incarcerated. As the weeks went by and the number of drink-free days grew, I began reflecting on the previous decade and decided to properly assess the damage. It was time to look beneath the hood and figure out exactly what was making the proverbial engine purr like an in-heat alley cat with an untreated dose of rabies. Did I drink because I was depressed or was I depressed because I drank? A conundrum that had held my brain captive for long enough until I eventually realised the truth – it didn't fucking matter.

First things first. I needed to wrap my head around the idea that addiction, like many things, is a vast spectrum and I had to figure out where I sat on that spectrum. At the risk of sounding trite, not all alcoholics look the same or act the same or even think about alcohol in the same way. I had to shake off the nonsensical 'one size fits all' approach that I subconsciously had when it came to viewing drink and drug addictions. For some it's strictly a numbing agent. For others it's a mood enhancer. For many it's a mixture of all the above. Everybody drinks differently. Even now, as somebody who is sober, I still have to keep an eye on myself when I notice myself judging or making assumptions about other alcoholics because their experiences are different from mine.

It didn't end there either. Before I started writing this book, I thought that alcohol was my only weakness. I didn't really think that cocaine was *too* much of a problem – I mean, I was aware that it wasn't exactly *not a problem*, but I viewed it more as the annoying know-it-all sidekick to the schoolyard bully, jeering over their shoulder in the playground, rather than being a true ringleader, right at the centre of proceedings, occupying the fortress of my mind and calling all the shots. Until I put myself under the microscope and thoroughly looked at the amount of cocaine I did, I deemed myself just another run-of-the-mill, line-snorting, session-going, pub-drinking dabbler. In reality, it was a little more serious than that.

A random example of its subtle omnipresence would be towards the end of Covid. My granny had called over for a glass of champagne with my mother to celebrate the closing ceremony of the pandemic (I think this was at some stage in 2020 ... *lol*). I joined them for the drink, got a bit giddy and immediately started sneaking upstairs throughout the evening to do bumps in the bathroom. Looking back, I think days like this were much more concerning than the big weekend sessions. At the time, I thought this was totally fine and recall even thinking to myself, 'Sure most people my age would be at this sort of craic if given the opportunity.' I might point out to you that this 'opportunity' was merely the chance to do cocaine in front of my mother and grandmother while sitting in the Dublin suburbs prematurely celebrating the end of a global pandemic that was only gathering momentum. It's not the same as going to space with Richard Branson or a free trip to the Maldives, is it? On another occasion around the same time, I was having a conversation with the parents of a close friend of mine at a small gathering in their home for his 30th. I was standing at the kitchen counter chatting to them when my nose started gushing blood. Before you say 'Oh, well, that could have been anything,' please bear in mind that it coincided with me practically breaking the sound barrier for the speed at which I was talking and pitching three different business ideas to them at once – so I'm pretty sure they knew what was happening. I think I blamed it on something ludicrous like the altitude. Because Clonskeagh is renowned for its height above sea level. For a long time, I also played the 'I only do drugs when I drink' card too. But soon enough, I was drinking just to have an excuse to do cocaine. Once the first pint was taken, I'd be off on the bag for the night. Particularly in the final few years, drinking without drugs became a messy, impatient and sloppy affair. I would search for the same rush of drugs via tequila shots and neat spirits but nothing would match the eye-opening electricity of a line of coke, and the pursuit of that energy would leave me in a complete stupor. So, yes, in short I think I had a cocaine problem.

As far as alcohol is concerned, on the grand spectrum of things I think I'm a fairly middle-of-the-road type of drunk. Could have been worse, could have been better. Due to various circumstances, notably my privilege, I never fully descended into the cartoon cliché of alcoholism, yet could never quite pull off a convincing performance of having a healthy relationship with the stuff either. On a few occasions, I was exposed to the new lows that forever lurked just beneath the surface – rock bottom is a fallacy, after all – and I slipped into red-eyed round-the-clock bingeing. I recall a period of a few weeks in 2021 when, after a particularly fraught series of arguments with my ex-girlfriend, I sequestered myself away in my mother's house while she was on holiday so I could drink in peace. I quickly slipped into the daily ritual of drinking a cup of red wine first thing in the morning, just to steady my nerves. Then I would have another cup to help me think straight. After that, I'd need one to cheer me up and one more to forget about the fighting. These morning settlers led to afternoons of tipping, before crossing over into a complete blackout in the night-time. When reality beckoned, due to a brief ceasefire in the relationship woes, I tried to taper off and slowly come back down from the week-long bender. But it wasn't that easy. I ended up taking to the bed for almost two days, mainlining anxiety and being too afraid to walk to the shops to buy cigarettes. I was trying to wean myself off the wine and catch up on my sleep, but every time I closed my eyes, a thousand images and voices would come screaming out of the shadows and cascade through my brain until I'd have a panic attack. This went on for about 18 hours, lying in the bed, skin sticky with cold sweat, twitching feet due to the anxiety and an open bottle of red wine on the bedside locker beside me. I'd intermittently wake up after fitful brushes of unconsciousness, reach for the bottle and swig from it, hoping that it would quieten my head sufficiently for me to fall back to sleep. What I could become, if presented with the opportunity. I never really thought it would ever get *that* bad and of course it didn't *stay* that bad either, but every time there was a spike of concentrated chaos in my life, a new level of alcoholism would be unlocked and I would graduate to uncharted territory and do something that I had never done before.

So there you have it. I'll leave it up to the professionals, armchair or otherwise, to decide which specific box to put me in, but for me it was clear that my drinking and use of cocaine were of a progressive and grave nature. The fear of returning to where I was is what spurred me on to go deeper into the mysterious abyss of sobriety, wading into the unknown while ignoring the daily instinct I had to press the self-destruct button and go back out drinking. It would have been very easy to do so. In truth, there were some people who thought I was taking things a bit too far by getting help. Some of my drinking friends thought it was all a bit over the top, this 'recovery' shite. I wasn't on skid row, after all. They would have preferred for me to just cut down on the all-nighters, lay off the cocaine and just go back to having a few casual pints on a Friday. I would have loved that too, but unfortunately that option had disappeared from the menu a long time ago. In the short term, I made the decision to cut myself off from a lot of people I used to drink with as the temptation would have been too much otherwise. Perhaps selfishly, I placed a large portion of my relationships under the guillotine of self-preservation and let the blade come down, decapitating my social life as I knew it. There wasn't any point in pretending that I could keep one foot in my old ways. Staying sober had to come first. If the changes weren't radical, I would never have stood a chance. I didn't realise it at the time, but these little acts would herald the very beginning of nurturing a real relationship with myself, understanding that I was entitled to boundaries and that it was okay to just say no to someone without a three-paragraph explanation or compromise. Too often in the past, I would lie when cancelling small plans for fear of letting someone down or worrying that it would result in them liking me less. Until recently, I thought that 'people pleasing' was just something done by a person who is excessively helpful with domestic chores and the like – doing the dishwasher, offering to help friends move furniture, etc. (Things I could never be accused of.) However, it's only in recovery that I learned that 'people pleasing' is actually when you feel such a strong urge to please others that you often ignore your own wants and needs, altering your personality to meet their approval. In hindsight, making that tiny gesture of separating myself from triggering places and people in the first few days of sobriety was the first in a series of acts of self-love that would eventually accumulate and help to change my life for ever. I won't pretend that it was easy or that at times I wasn't lonely. For the first few months, I was just about clinging on by my fingertips. Here is an example of my average day-to-day at the beginning, just to give you an idea of what it entailed:

- wake up
- smoke three cigarettes
- go for a walk
- smoke more cigarettes
- text some alcoholics
- try to write jokes in the notes section of my iPhone
- plan the podcast
- wonder will I ever experience the sensation of joy again
- watch porn
- more cigarettes
- argue with girlfriend
- episode of *Bake Off*
- cigarettes
- bed

A lot has changed since then, and not just the cigarettes. I'd like to think I'm a little less selfish, too. In the first month or so of recovery, I made a good friend with another alcoholic called Paul. Paul and myself had got sober at the same time, and we shared a similar type of bond to the one that you have with a stranger in an airport when you're both enduring the endless torture of waiting for the same delayed flight. You find yourselves bound by circumstance and connected through experiencing the ordeal together. Having somebody else in the same boat as me helped alleviate those messy emotions of the early days. We would play bad golf together, having good conversations about how things used to be, how we were feeling that morning and then how we planned on navigating our way through the remainder of the week. It was as if we were two teenage boys figuring out how to be adults for the first time and learning how to live in a world beyond our comprehension. After the golf, we would drive home and I would become very depressed. No amount of Marlboro Lights or jellies from Centra could generate the same high as a casual few pints, and it would take a long time to rewire the internal reward system my brain had become accustomed to; since I was 18 every emotion, feeling or mood that I either liked or didn't like was enhanced or softened with the promise of a drink or a drug.

Until I got sober, my life was no more than a series of infinite transactions.

But somehow, I did what I was told, I didn't drink and slowly but surely, things began to get better.

The clouds didn't lift entirely but every now and then they would part enough for me to feel a sense of optimism and say to myself 'You're doing okay, Mark, you're doing okay. Just hang in there.' I continued with the podcast; my fans helped keep the wolf from the door via subscriptions to my Patreon account for bonus content (of which there was very little). I also landed a scriptwriting job for a gaming commercial in the UK and Asia which helped keep me out of the red. I was desperately trying to piece back together the trajectory I'd had two years previously and regenerate a bit of momentum.

One afternoon I got a call from the Sugar Club in Dublin who wanted to book me for a live show. It transcended all logic as to why they wanted me for a gig because at that point, my presence on the internet was about as reliable as the temperament of a GP's receptionist. I had also been on stage approximately zero times in my life and as somebody who had a generalised anxiety disorder which occasionally manifested in social anxiety and irrational fears such as getting on aeroplanes or public speaking, of course I said yes. The show was not going to be until March and it was now early December, so

I didn't need to worry about it for a few months anyway. It was a tomorrow problem. As far as I was concerned, my life was already in complete disarray anyway – why not throw in another curveball? The day the tickets went on sale, I was extraordinarily nervous. Due to the erratic nature of my social media activity and irregular podcast recordings, it was impossible to know if the listeners were still listening. The tickets sold out in eight minutes. I couldn't believe it. I stood in my bedroom with tears in my eyes. We immediately added another date and that sold out too. And then a third. Three sold-out nights at the Sugar Club for my debut. Absolutely magic. None of those people knew that I was in recovery or were aware of the shit that I was going through at the time. Everybody has their own shit too and *nobody is thinking about you as much as you are thinking about you,* after all. What people don't realise is that each person who bought a ticket that day had effectively handed me a torch and given me enough light to make my way out of the dark tunnel that my drinking had brought me down.

In the months building up to the gigs, aside from the expected levels of self-doubt and apprehension, I started to realise that these shows were definitely going to happen and soon I would be standing on stage in front of hundreds of people without a drink in my hand or a drug in my system. This was already beyond what I ever could have expected from recovery. Truthfully, I never thought my career would make it to the stage, such was the extent of my anxiety. This marked the beginning of a new chapter in my life that I never could have anticipated – the birth of hope. Things were happening that I had always deemed unthinkable. Crafting a 90-minute stand-up special was literally a dream come true, something I had wanted to do since I first watched *Politics* by Ricky Gervais on my video iPod at the age of 14.

Recovery was teaching me that it was okay to believe in myself and pursue my dreams. Self-belief was different from the fragile, conceited arrogance that I used to know, which was permanently underpinned by crippling insecurity and fear. I realised that if I just didn't drink I would potentially grow into a person I would be happy to call *myself*. It was tough not experiencing the manic highs that I was used to with booze, but I certainly enjoyed the safety from its subsequent wicked lows. With every month of clean time under my belt, and a gathering sense of consistency, I started to realise that maybe I wasn't the worst person in the world and perhaps I was just wired a bit differently. I started learning that most of my issues are ultimately rooted in a fundamental lack of self-worth and an oversupply of fear. But by doing the next right thing – trying to help others and following other practices that were suggested to me by more serene individuals – every day I would feel a little bit better about the future and have less of a desire not to be *me*. Putting the drink down would mark the first, tiny opening of a door of self discovery, even if only by a crack, enough to stick my toe in, and afforded me the chance to observe the way I think and to establish that there is a difference between my *self* and my *thoughts*.

Today I believe that I am worth more than the consequences of bringing a drink to my lips. In this current 24-hour period, I can see that I deserve better than the misery and uncertainty that awaits me at the bottom of a glass. I do not know if I will ever drink again. *Never is a very dangerous word.*

In March 2022, I walked onto the stage of the Sugar Club to a sea of nearly three hundred people, clapping their hands and calling my name. Some of them were definitely on cocaine. I was nearly six months sober and it was the most terrifying moment of my life. But I wasn't thinking about a drink.

What I could become, if presented with the opportunity.

CHAPTER 10

MEDICATE OR MEDITATE

Happiness is our true nature, our essential being. The transient happiness that we seem to derive from external experiences actually arises only from within ourself, and is experienced by us due to the temporary calming of our mind that occurs whenever any of our desires are fulfilled. So long as our mind is extroverted, attending to anything other than our own essential self-conscious being, we can never experience perfect, permanent and unqualified happiness.
– *Bhagavan Sri Ramana Maharshi*

If I say too much now, I'll feel like a fraud.

Throughout my years of drinking, I actively baulked at the notion of living on any sort of spiritual plane. In truth, I was sceptical of any person who professed to derive meaning from any department of life other than alcohol, sex, relationships, art, greed or substances. They were either lying or freaks. Just like my juvenile preconception of what an alcoholic looked like, my idea of a spiritual individual also stemmed from the schoolyard. I bought into the myth that everybody who derives meaning through spiritual ways – religious or otherwise – was somehow intellectually inferior to the rest of us and deserved to be scorned. In my eyes, if you were spiritual, it meant that you were either a religious wack job or an acid-dropping hippie. There was never any in between; my prejudice allowed for very little nuance. Through all my drinking years, I ran in the opposite direction from any conversations surrounding real philosophy. In my nihilistic delusion, I genuinely believed that I drank because I was more aware of life's meaninglessness than most and simply chose to escape in order to distract myself from the truth. Aside from being concerningly insane and frightfully arrogant, it was also total nonsense. Pretentious, un-deep *16-year-old-after-two-puffs-of-a-joint-with-a-tattered-copy-of-The-Catcher-in-the-Rye-under-his-arm* levels of pseudo-cynicism, deployed purely because it was easier than asking myself any of the tougher questions.

Getting sober was a humbling odyssey into the unknown and I realised quickly that the happiest people I knew seemed to be the ones who engaged in a regular spiritual practice. Just because I was no longer filling the void with booze and drugs, it didn't mean that the void no longer needed filling. Performing the emotional Heimlich manoeuvre on my life that was getting sober cleared the road of many of the closed-minded preconceptions I had had about belief systems and I became a lot more receptive to the idea of tending to my *inner garden* and looking at the world within. (I know!)

The first few months of my sobriety had really forced me to evaluate how I derived meaning from life in the first place. The further away from booze I walked, the more clearly I could see the power of its grip. Every decision, every relationship, every holiday, every job had been influenced by it in some shape or form and the extent of its infiltration was truly mind-blowing. There wasn't a corner of my life untouched by its meddling paws. For instance, I realised then that I was 30 years of age and I didn't have a single hobby. I met only the oldest of my friends away from bars and pubs, in non-drinking environments. I genuinely didn't see people sober. Without getting too lofty, I had to sift through the contents of my character and figure out which parts of me were *me* and which parts were just offshoots of the culture that had imbued my entire being. To put it simply, I had to put down the pints and ask myself who I was. Without the pubs and the clubs and the bars and the wine – what was left? That process is still ongoing, by the way.

It was then that I started learning about what I have been referring to as self myths. Here are some straightforward examples of the myths that I had previously maintained about my character and the type of guy that I was. For every one of these self myths that I went on to debunk, I was one step closer to figuring out who I wasn't – and that seemed like a decent enough starting point before undertaking the much larger, complicated mission of figuring out who I wanted to be. Learning to ask these simple questions about myself was transformative and the beginning of an overall willingness to change absolutely everything about my life. I still try to do it as often as possible; ask myself is this a myth or is this reality? For instance:

MYTH:

I like to go to the theatre because I am a cultured man.

REALITY:

I enjoy drinking two bottles of red wine while criticising the performances of the actors on stage and fantasising about how many Oscars I would have won if I had chosen to tread the boards.

MYTH:

I much prefer city breaks to beach holidays. I am a city person and that will always be the case.

REALITY:

I enjoy drinking and cities seem to provide the most options when it comes to places I can drink.

If I go somewhere far away from a city I might be forced to participate in an activity like swimming in the sea or climbing up a mountain and that will make me want to shoot myself in the face. I would prefer to be drinking.

MYTH:

I am the type of guy who enjoys going to a cosy little pub with a novel and having a quiet pint; it's much more wholesome than other types of drinking.

REALITY:

I like drinking everywhere, at all times, every day with anybody. Quiet pints. Loud pints. Christmas pints. Funeral pints. It doesn't matter. And I haven't read a novel since secondary school.

MYTH:

I like going on dates, they're a great way of connecting with people and discovering interesting new places to eat in the city.

REALITY:

I enjoy getting shitfaced with enthusiastic strangers. It gives me the opportunity to perform, to say a lot while saying very little, and I never have to see them again.

I could go on listing myths ad infinitum. I am still only at the discovery stage when it comes to exploring the never-ending number of fables and stories that I had previously told myself about the type of person that I was. It will take a long time to change all of that. I couldn't believe it but I had spent my whole life putting myself into little boxes, telling myself things like 'You're not the type of person who does X' or 'You wouldn't be able for Y' or 'You're the sort of guy who thinks this' or 'You don't like things like that.' All of it was complete bullshit.

As time went on, I became more steadfast in my decision to stay in recovery and the knowledge that it was clearly the right thing to do – I was already gaining a deeper understanding of myself – but as many alcoholics had correctly warned, staying away from the booze would only do so much in thoroughly satisfying my mind. If I really wanted to get better, there would need to be a deeper, inner contentment, a connection to something greater than myself. Otherwise I would almost certainly drink again. In the very beginning, I enjoyed the yawning, sleepy peace of no longer causing chaos on a weekly basis, but soon the soul started calling out for more. You cannot bring a wild animal in from the cold and expect it to tame itself, however nice the house is. At the very least it will piss on the floor and at worst it might tear your face off. My addictions were capable of doing both. (I'm slightly uncomfortable with that metaphor because it makes it sound like I am referring to myself as a wild animal while also boasting about how nice my house is, and neither of those points is what I intended. I do think there is something deeply unsettling about men comparing them-selves to tigers and lions anyway, as it's usually only done by incredibly musclebound morons with bleached teeth and tribal tattoos promoting online coaching businesses.)

Wanting to dip my toe in the waters of self-work but without any knowledge of where the bloody water was, I called again on the advice of *the most outrageous man* who had laughed down the phone at me a few months before. Aside from acting as my personal therapist, close friend and mentor, he was also more than happy to come on board as my spiritual concierge too. A simple practice that he encouraged me to adopt in these early stages of recovery was to start writing gratitude lists. Get out of my head and start getting grateful. It seemed silly at first. *Ten things every day that you are grateful for.* I'm not *Lovin' Dublin*, for fuck's sake. Even in recovery it seemed that I couldn't escape the never-ending culture of list-making that our society has become. I also considered myself allergic to words like 'gratitude', associating them only with the bland lexicon of phoney wellness bloggers or American celebrities. *It's very easy to be grateful when you're earning 20 million dollars a movie, Mr ... The Rock.* My outlook was so cynical, I always assumed the worst in everything and I probably would have placed the word 'gratitude' in the same bracket as 'toxic' or 'gaslighting'; words that originally meant something serious, but having been bastardised by gobshites on the internet were slowly losing their value. Fortunately, I managed to do the right thing, which again was the direct opposite of what my head was telling me. And so, I started writing gratitude lists. Ten things every day, ranging from the mundane to the insane, and occasionally including the extraordinary. As far as I can tell, the benefit of these lists, like most of the spiritual practices that I would later try to adopt, is that they dragged me away from the recesses of my mind and forced me to shake off the permanent coat of self-pity and *poor me*'s that I wore every day in early recovery. By rooting me in the present they were like a splash of cold water to the face, reminding me about the *grand scheme of things* and protecting me from my habitual tendency to slip off into fantasy land, where my wants will always surpass my needs and relapse lurks behind every corner. I now have any number of these lists that I can look back on and revisit, reflecting on where I was emotionally on any given day and realising that in hindsight, most of my problems or worries never seem to be as big as they felt at the time.

Somebody said to me once, 'It's okay to look back on the past, but don't fucking stare!' and that helped me enormously. Reading over the old lists can sometimes be tough but that is just the nature of recovery, if not the nature of life, in all of its confusing, bizarre and non-linear beauty. Against my better judgement, I've included a few lists of my own for you to take a look at. There is nothing particularly profound about these lists and in all honesty I had to resist the urge to alter them and make my mornings seem more insightful or inspired, but the reality is that mundanity is what I had craved throughout my latter years of drinking, and it is the simple things like a morning coffee, watching the sun come up or having a good chat with a friend that to me are the true gifts of recovery.

29/04/22
This morning I am grateful for:

1. Waking up in London sober.
2. Performing the show tonight to fans of the podcast.
3. Repairing my relationship with the city of London and knowing it can be a happy place again.
4. Kind messages on Instagram from people coming to the show tonight.
5. Connections with Craig and making peace with the past.
6. Spending time with my brother Freddie and him getting to see me on stage.

7. Enjoying my time in London, happy and healthy and doing live comedy.
8. Moving on from the past and living in the present.
9. Beautiful weather.
10. A relaxing sober travel day yesterday, everything is so much easier when not drinking my way through the airport.

25/05/22
This morning I am grateful for:

1. Going easier on myself and remembering I'm doing my best in recovery.
2. Solid writing time on the computer. At least one hour every day.
3. Replying to texts when I get them.
4. More accepting of a life without booze, this life will be better for me in the long run.
5. Reaching out to people when feeling lonely or disconnected.
6. Understanding that some people will not wish to engage in certain conversations about the past and that's okay.
7. Trying to be kind. Doing something nice for someone else. Things are getting better.

8. Knowing I deserve to be happy.
9. Drinking more water. Trying to smoke a little less.
10. Reaching out to someone else I haven't spoken to in ages.

26/07/22
This morning I am grateful for:

1. Growth in my communication due to recovery.
2. Less black-and-white thinking (sometimes).
3. A walk on the pier to start the day.
4. A chat with R this morning.
5. Knowing that I have wonderful, real, honest connections in recovery that are solely built on love and support.
6. The warm weather.
7. Hearing about the good news K got.
8. Beginning my day with gratitude reminds me of how lucky I am to be here sober.
9. Rigorous honesty.
10. Buying flowers for the apartment.

My diligence as a spiritual aspirant definitely fluctuates and some days are better than others. I don't always find the time to write out my lists and oftentimes the best I can do is wheel out a Top Five with the believable conviction of a teenager (me) rattling off the names of fictional girls he's kissed on holiday.

In the summer of 2022, I think I had a spiritual awakening. Well, something along those lines, anyway. Perhaps it was a nervous breakdown. Either way, I was seven or eight months sober and the relationship I was in had finally ended. I found myself alone, living in Dún Laoghaire and doing my best to avoid pressing the big red self-destruct button that hovered tantalisingly beneath my fingertips. Every single day it increased in size. I had spent the previous few months dissociating from my old life but had yet to cultivate or nurture a new one. All of my eggs had been split between two baskets; my recovery and my relationship. It felt like each one was responsible for keeping the other intact. Of course that wasn't tenable. Going through a break-up sober was almost surreal in its agony. A root canal without the anaesthetic. I had nowhere to run with the pain and I found myself at a crossroads. One foot in a new life; in a world of gratitude lists, honest human connection and trying to improve on the person that I once was.

But then the other foot; forever stuck floating over my old life, eagerly awaiting the chance to step right back into the manic internal destruction that was how things used to be. It was touch and go, to be honest.

At so many intervals around those few weeks I came within inches of closing the curtains, ordering a bag and sending myself into oblivion for a few days. I had it all mapped out. *What was the point in recovering if things were going to go to shit, anyway?* I was still under the hilariously misguided impression that no longer drinking would mean a straight swap into a life of tranquillity and peace, that somehow I'd be able to swerve pain and dodge anguish as long as I stayed dry. The aforementioned transactional outlook on life was hard to shake off, as you can see. Life on life's terms meant experiencing everything sober – the good, the bad and the break-ups. The whole proverbial shooting match.

Acceptance is the answer to all my problems today. Coming to terms with the fact that I would still be a flawed human being even in recovery, with all my cracks and weaknesses, ugly feelings and bad days, anxieties and panic attacks, shortcomings and oddities, marked a significant turning point in my journey of sobriety. Once I started to accept that life would still be life, and things would still be messy – people are inherently messy – I could start making progress in my recovery. This was the realest way of living I had ever known. A by-product of accepting life on life's terms was that I began to see the value in accepting myself for who I am. Not punishing myself for who I am not.

Fortunately, between fistfuls of Haribo and chain-smoking cigarettes on my balcony, I made the wise decision to contact another alcoholic and ask him for his advice about how to handle life after a break-up in sobriety. He told me to try doubling up on my meditations. There wasn't anything to double up on. I hadn't meditated since secondary school when we were sent on a religious retreat, and even then they had to cancel the group meditation halfway through because one student had tried too hard to fart loudly and had ended up shitting himself. (And I'd do it again.) I explained to him that I was a complete beginner when it came to meditating and that I wouldn't really know where to start, but he reassured me that by simply expressing a desire to meditate and an openness to the practice of it I was already halfway there. He then gave me the name of an app (Insight Timer) and sent me over a couple of guided meditations that he thought might be useful for me to start with, given my current state of inner affairs. (These were Sarah Blondin's 'The Power in Letting Go' and 'Learning to Surrender'.) The first time I tried to do it, I went down to Dún Laoghaire pier and after about 30 seconds I became convinced that an old man was laughing at me, so I faked a phone call and got the hell out of there. I walked home red-faced, as if I'd been caught wanking behind the rocks. *Eckhart Tolle never had to put up with this shit*, I thought.

On the second day I tried it again and this time I found myself feeling that something significant had occurred – it was as if there was a powerful shift in my psyche and a change in the way I was viewing the world. Even if only for a moment. I was almost emotional. I remember it so vividly. I was lying on my back on the right side of the East Pier, down by the bandstand. The weather was glorious. I spent five or ten minutes staring intently at the horizon, focusing on my breath, with my back arched and my lungs open wide, allowing each inhale and exhale to consume my mind, slowly letting all the feelings and emotions wash over me – but for once I wasn't resisting them or trying to redirect my thoughts towards a calmer or happier place. Out of the blue, I was overcome with a hazy sense of calm and it was there that I surrendered once again. To my recovery. To a new way of life. To the fact that my relationship was over and that I was simply going to have to process the pain rather than bury it or deny it. I had nowhere to go with it. I was sad but I was here, clear-headed and alive. Sitting by the water, feeling the cool stone on the back of my legs and the salty air on my face, I knew that I was finally experiencing a vital element of the human experience, unsedated, as myself. I was *awake*. There was a profound and moving beauty to the pain I felt that day because I knew it to be true and that I could trust it. There was nothing synthetic about what I was feeling, which was totally different from my previous life. I didn't deploy the usual coping mechanism of relying on anger or contrived detachment to see me through the initial days of pain. I was suffering and that was okay.

Those early meditations marked a significant turning point in several arenas of my life:

my recovery; my spirituality; and particularly my day-to-day dealings with anxiety and panic attacks. I was slowly learning the art of allowing feelings to happen without always needing to fight them off. It was okay to put down the stick and let myself be angry, upset, frustrated or afraid. *It would always pass.* So much of the inner turmoil that had been present for the duration of my childhood, adolescence, teenage years and then into adulthood had been born out of, and amplified by, trying to combat how I felt and overcome any uncomfortable emotions rather than sitting with them. 'Don't feel like that', 'Don't go in there like that', 'Don't be anxious', 'Don't let people know you're unhappy', 'Don't let that get to you', 'Don't be such an idiot.' For a man who spoke so much, I realised then that I was almost entirely taciturn when it came to assertive emotional expression. Once I started meditating, I discovered the power of letting go, accepting things for how they were and resisting the constant urge to go to war with my emotions, in a lose–lose boxing match. Now don't get me wrong, just because I fleetingly witnessed the transformative power of meditation, it doesn't mean that I was able to bottle it, capture it and figure out how to apply that feeling to my personal life whenever I needed to. If that was the case, I would still be on the pier now, like a human-sized Xanax bar, staring into the sun with a smile on my face. No, the feeling didn't stay for very long. I was still smoking two cigarettes per meditation and checking my phone at least once. Nothing changed overnight, but at least I had been given a glimpse of what was possible. And now I wanted more.

I'm not academically minded, nor am I remotely informed on the subject of meditation, matters of the *self* or any other complex spiritual concepts that are definitely out of my reach intellectually, but I might just offer that by bringing myself somewhere quiet, getting still and breathing for about 15 minutes every day, I was soon, for the first time in my life, beginning to feel connected to something much greater than myself. It was remarkable.

The simple practice of deep breathing and focusing on the 'now' resulted in a lifting of the spirit, even if my mood was still low, and a quietening of the mind unlike anything else.

A good friend of mine, Theo, who is considerably more wise and connected than I am, had
been prodding me with the task of separating
myself from my thoughts for quite a while now.
Initially, I thought it was a load of bollocks and
accused him of being insane. How could I *be*
anything other than my thoughts? He was absolutely correct, though – it *is* possible to observe
one's own thoughts. With a bit of practice, during
my own little meditations, I was slowly able to
sit back and watch the thoughts come past me,
like clouds floating by, shapeless and incomplete,
without judgement or intervention. This resulted
in experiencing an inner quiet that alleviated the
manic temptation to fuck my entire life up during
the days of the break-up, soothing me on a deeply
primal level and eliminating the near-constant
desire to be somewhere else. By sitting still and
not doing anything, good stuff was happening. I
didn't turn into Henry Sugar or see the light, and I
definitely snapped out of it quicker than your tight
friend could ask if there's a free bar at a wedding,
but there were momentary breakthroughs in
those meditative states that either switched on a
light somewhere inside me or turned one off. 'I
am not my thoughts' quickly became a powerful

mantra for me to use when dealing with anxiety, irrational fears, panic attacks and general negative self-talk. When thoughts like 'Fuck everybody, I'm going drinking' resurfaced during feelings of anger or frustration, I was able to identify them as separate from me, and not a reflection of my failing at recovery or what I intrinsically believed to be best for myself in that moment. Ever since, I try to judge myself as little as possible for the thoughts that come into my head. I urge you to do the same. For example, if you see an old woman crossing the street and you immediately wonder what would happen if she fell in front of a bus, it doesn't make you a bad person. Now, if you then toss a Werther's Original out in front of the 46A like fishing bait, but for pensioners, then maybe you need a bit of help. In all seriousness, though, the result of judging myself less for the thoughts that pass through my head has been a breakthrough. I used to punish myself ferociously for the things I thought, at times even convincing myself that I was a bad person due to their inexplicable nature. Letting go of those ridiculous expectations that my brain should be constantly working a certain way has been tremendously beneficial for my overall sense of self-love. I have also found it liberating to laugh at my own thinking, at just how crazy it can be sometimes. When practised (and *only* when practised regularly) this massively diminishes my tendency to spiral into streams of negativity, particularly when I feel cornered, trapped, threatened or afraid.

I once heard an addict say that he doesn't go sea swimming because he 'didn't do *that* much cocaine' and it's still one of the funniest things that I have ever heard. Like him, I didn't start flinging myself into the sea after a brief foray into mindfulness, but I was certainly more open to trying new things. The results of meditating had been so instant and so obvious that I was amazed it had never been prescribed to me in the past. It was certainly the most rigorously transformative act in terms of combating anxiety. It opened up my eyes to a universe of self-work that I knew nothing about and shattered all of my preconceptions about spirituality, breathwork and the very essence of *being*. I wondered what else I had missed out on throughout the years of gallivanting.

Without the usual rules and limitations when it came to how I looked at the world, I found myself feeling very open and awake – on a brand new journey – slowly discovering who I was. There were lots of trial and lots of error, but because I wasn't burying my feelings in the bottom of a bag or on three-day benders any more, I was a lot less anxious and rigid in the way I expressed my emotions, and I slowly became better at isolating and understanding particular feelings whenever they came up. All of a sudden I started to feel a little bit of compassion for my former self, too. Perhaps I wasn't the worst in the world, ever? Maybe I was a sick person trying to get well rather than a bad person trying to become good or a broken person trying to become fixed. I didn't hate the face I saw in the mirror any more and I even sympathised with my body for treating it the way I had over the years. It was a strange, cathartic and beautiful stage of my recovery, where I learned the importance of having a relationship with myself.

A couple of weeks later, I found myself on Killiney Beach on a Friday night with two new friends, Stef and Laura, who had kindly taken me under their wing after the break-up, to attend some form of full moon ceremony that would include healing, reiki, chanting and manifesting. It read like an East London Tinder bio. If you had told me on that awful night many years before when I was sneaking bags of cocaine across the Irish Sea in the ripped seam of my North Face jacket that I would one day be doing the downward-facing dog on Killiney Beach with five hundred strangers and not feeling like a complete pervert ... Well, I probably would have believed you, actually. I mean, I *was* high on cocaine after all.

I used to think that *self-love* just meant buying an expensive item of clothing I couldn't afford or blowing off the regular diet and adopting the eating habits of a 64-year-old polo-wearing cruise ship passenger from Arkansas on the retirement trip of a lifetime. Little did I know that the greatest acts of self-love are the seemingly insignificant ones, the tiny patterns of personal improvement that quietly enhanced my spiritual condition and overall sense of self-esteem. Throughout my addiction, I was only used to huge, sweeping dramatic gestures and was forever making all-or-nothing promises without any follow-through or commitment. I had no idea that usually the most authentic growth in life happens on an incremental basis rather than overnight. Self-love was choosing to do the right thing for myself again and again and again. The beauty lay in the consistency. One day at a time. The best way for me to observe and monitor if and how much I am recovering is to pay attention to my reaction when something challenging happens in life. If I respond differently from the way I would have in the past, with my words and in my actions, then I am breaking the cycle and that in itself is an act of self-love, healing and growth. Interrupting my own thoughts when I feel myself slipping into a negative spiral and whispering 'You are loved' is an act of self-love.

Oh and by the way, you are loved.

Everything in you that you don't need, you can let go of.

You don't need loneliness for you couldn't possibly be alone. You don't need greed because you already have it all.

Ram Dass

− Jon Hopkins, 'Sit Around the Fire'

CHAPTER 11

HOW ARE YOUR HEARTS? HOW ARE YOUR HEADS?

Alas, you can't spend *all* your time meditating on the end of Dún Laoghaire pier, trying to see the light. Once the summer passed, it grew a tad bit repetitive and, let's be honest, cold. In lieu of licking toads or booking myself in for a cacao ceremony (that will be the second book) I felt it was high time I started living. I was just shy of one year dry, the autumn leaves were falling and I found myself suffering from an unwanted sense of limbo and unease. I knew that I was doing the right thing by staying sober but resented how seemingly *quiet and boring* my life had become. All the gushing, engulfing serenity of those water-side meditations did little to abate the sense of solitude that came from my newfound existence. I often found myself at home alone on Saturday nights, staring at the walls and waiting for the phone to ring. I was sick of meeting married friends for coffee at 9.30 on a Sunday morning and for that to count as my social activity for the weekend. Being single in your thirties can be isolating. Being single and sober in your thirties was even more complicated. The realisations pricked and irritated like bee stings at how little 'life' I had left once the booze was gone. I expected a big life of exhilarating brilliance in sobriety, but this one spelled seclusion and sadness. At times it felt like I was existing just below *life* or watching it happen over my head, almost as if I was trapped in a frozen pond and looking up at the people above walking by. *Poor me, poor me ... pour me a drink.* Self-pity is addictive in itself. The long and short of it is that when I was partying, the weekends took care of themselves and all my socialising automatically fell into place. I never really had to make plans. When in need of stimulation, I would simply launch out a message into a few WhatsApp groups and the night out would unfold. Relationships in recovery would require a lot more work, more nurturing and upkeep.

In the end, I had become so preoccupied in feeling sorry for myself that I almost missed the glaring punch-in-the-face obviousness of my predicament – I was still totally imprisoned by my own thinking. I was so wrapped up and consumed by the fact that life wasn't unfolding the way I thought it would that I had essentially walked myself into a cell of preconceptions about what recovery looked like, placed my hands inside the arms of a straitjacket, tied the knot and swallowed the key.

The prison bars trapping me now were the limitless rules and expectations that my ego had maintained about how things *should* work.

Things should be a certain way. Everything was a transaction, after all. Unless I ditched these staunch delusions and shook the tree from its roots, I would be destined for a life of solitary unhappiness, whether I was with people or not. Now that I had removed alcohol from my life, I had given myself an honest chance at discovering real purpose, but it was still just a chance. The only thing standing between myself and a life beyond my wildest dreams was me. But I had to go out there and live it – and that very often required doing the exact opposite of what my brain tells me to do. Writing this book was one of those things. The biggest threat to me are my thoughts and if I can just *get out of my own way*, contentment and enlightenment are available in abundance.

In any case, back to the real world. In order to survive *out there*, I would require people. And those people tend to be in places. And those people who go to places often like to do things. And all of those things were terrifying. Reality is ugly and loud and unbearably bad-mannered. But it had to be done. If I wanted a stimulating existence that stretched beyond the walls of Dún Laoghaire, I would have to stop banging my head against the brick wall of fear and force myself to look at what was on the other side. Life will always find a way of interfering with my expectations about how things will unfold, revealing that true change only ever occurs if things are done differently from how they were done before. My liberation lies in doing the opposite of what my head tells me to. Or, to put it even more simply, in the words of Michael Scott: 'You should never settle for who you are.'

Over the next few months, I set about challenging my preconceptions about sober life – what I was capable of, what I could enjoy – and attempted to debunk the numerous self-propagated myths I had held about living *on the dry*, embarking on a once-in-a-lifetime voyage into the uncharted waters of life, with the sun on my face, the wind at my back and no longer asleep at the wheel.

MYTH:

My friends won't like me if I am sober and boring.

REALITY:

The allure to adopt the demeanour of a wounded hero returning from war and accuse friends of deserting me was very enticing at times at the beginning, which is *deeply* ironic, as I was the one who went AWOL. With time, I've learned that it's only natural for some friendships to fall away after a great change. And let's be honest, if one of my friends got massively into an obscure hobby like horse riding and started talking incessantly about horse-related stuff, wearing jodhpurs into cafés and using one of those little whip things to smack me on the bottom whenever I walked too slow, I would probably keep my distance from him, too.

I understand now that it's okay to move on from relationships in life and that it's not necessarily an ill reflection of the other person or of me. Getting sober does not merit canonisation – everybody has their own version of a Sunday night comedown and unwanted aspects of life that they have to wrap their heads around. I wasn't the first person to stare at the grey London sky of a Monday morning or scan the empty expressions of commuters on the Tube and wonder what it's really all about. People grow in different directions; and some friendships thrive in multiple contexts while others only thrive in one. I think of it in the same way I would a holiday romance. Throughout my twenties, I always felt a compulsion to preserve friendships for too long because I was worried that if they fizzled out it was indicative of a failing on my part or that I wasn't good enough for them. It was much easier to maintain a vague thread of contact and launch out non-committal text messages every four months about maybe meeting up soon, only to stare at the screen for a few minutes and hope that the other person wouldn't reply rather than accepting the fact that we were just moving away from each other. It's not like that any more.

The friendships I have now – a mixture of old and new – are honest, upfront and non-transactional. I've become a better friend to the people I love and am also more careful over who I decide to let into my life. For once, I can pick up the phone and call Stuart; I can be there for him when he needs me. I can shut up and listen. Every family event doesn't need to revolve around me. I can make promises to people and stick to them. I've got my dignity back. Back when I was drinking, I carried so much guilt about being a bad friend, brother, son, colleague, partner and person that I didn't really believe I deserved any boundaries. I would sometimes allow myself to be mistreated and exploited by others, as I thought it was a fair punishment for my own momentary lapses in moral judgement over the years. In early sobriety, I struggled to adapt to the transition from regularly texting almost 50 people at any given time, to suddenly texting about four. Other alcoholics would pacify me and gently say, 'Mark, you've got to give time, *time*,' and that's probably the most vital, albeit unwanted, advice that I have ever received on this journey. As soon as I put down the drink, I expected everything to happen at once in my social life. Before I even identified what it was I wanted, I was cursing sobriety for not delivering it.

I spent a lot of time wandering down cul-de-sacs of old behaviours, searching for answers in the very same places that had forced me to ask the questions.

At times, I even tried adopting the same social habits as before I stopped drinking, but going to pubs wasn't exactly recommended in early recovery; and, in my experience, watching other people do cocaine is like watching other people do karaoke – unless you're directly involved in the activity yourself, it immediately becomes the most infuriating spectacle of stupidity that you've ever witnessed. Nowadays, there are about 10 people in my inbox on any given day, and I would go to the end of the earth for each of them.

It's important for me to remember that pulling a dramatic U-turn on my life probably came as a bit of a shock to some. Old friends might find it hard to believe that I no longer enjoy the music when at times I was the one conducting the orchestra. Some people get a bit awkward about recovery too, and that's normal. It's probably hard to know how bad it got. There is no polite way of gauging, either. Their eyes tend to just linger over yours a little longer after you've told them, in case you might give it away with a wrinkle on your forehead or a chip in your tooth. *Did he like the occasional glass of sherry after lunch or was he drinking shots of Domestos out of a sandwich bag before doing the school run? Did he sneak in an extra pint without telling the wife or was he hiding naggins up his bum going through airport security?* I often found myself telling people that I was an alcoholic but immediately following up with a self-deprecatory joke about how I wasn't that bad, just to reassure them that I am still normal and I'm still one of them. But of course, I was *never* one of them. I've now stopped making those jokes. I'm happy enough with the person I'm becoming, and if there's one thing I have learned over the years, it's that people are going to think whatever they want to think, regardless of what I tell them. Trying to control another person's perception of me is as futile as my attempts to have *four casual pints.*

MYTH:

I will never be able to date again now that I am sober.

REALITY:

If there is one surefire way to cut down on the trivial, repetitive and meaningless dating of modern life, it's giving up the booze. Four hours with a stranger suddenly feels like a fucking marathon once you don't have the lubricating conviviality of alcohol to rely on.

When I stopped drinking, I quickly became a lot more selective when it came to dating strangers from the internet. And when I say selective, of course I mean *afraid.* It's hard to believe that even matters of the primal variety were so heavily influenced by booze, but at this point nothing would shock me. As it would transpire, I have only ever been on one sober first date in recovery and that was with my current girl-friend, Doireann. I always find it weird when people say 'my *current* girlfriend'. It suggests a transience, almost as if they're approaching their best before date or they know that they're on the way out. Or perhaps they're sitting at some sort of girlfriend version of YO! Sushi and there is constant flow of girlfriends coming out of the little hole, rotating slowly along the conveyor belt, and this particular girlfriend just happens to be the *current* one.

The first time I went on a date with Doireann was in early November 2022. We spent two hours walking around Sandycove, up through Dalkey village and then back down to Dún Laoghaire. At the time, I was just over one year sober and it had been the hardest year of my life. But she didn't know any of that yet. I met her on the road near my house. She got out of her car in the rain, we went for a cup of tea in my apartment and I knew I loved her. She was as ethereal as my recollection is cliché. I've learned things about love from her that I could have spent 10 lifetimes trying to figure out. I am blessed to have her in my life and I adore the ground she walks on. If I could borrow the way she looks at the world, I would almost certainly be a happier man.

MYTH:

I will never feel the connection that I used to do when drinking and doing drugs with people.

REALITY:

I enjoyed the sense of connection that came from that, of course I did. And occasionally I miss the camaraderie of going to the pub with my friends. I miss standing over a house key and a bag in the cramped cubicle of a pub toilet, whispering furiously to my temporary mate. I'm only human.

I often find myself yearning for that *extra* feeling, the elusive sensation I spent the whole of my twenties chasing – when you're six drinks in and it feels like anything could happen or when you have the first sip of a beer on holiday, the one after a long day in the sun, and you've got fresh clothes on with the prickly remnants of the sea and sun cream stuck to your skin. What a sense of opportunity it brought! One drink in and I would finally remember that I had my whole life ahead of me. The shoulders would relax, the foot would cease tapping. I certainly miss the warm, delicious embrace of a bottle of red wine in the winter too and there's a reason I attached myself to its hip for so long. I am no denouncer of the wonders of alcohol. I'm grateful for a lot of the experiences it brought me, I'm just ready to close that chapter of my life and pursue value elsewhere. Well ... I didn't really have a choice, did I?

In short, yes, life can be exhausting when you're *awake* all the time – and at times that's what it feels like – it can be a bit of a slog. But what I've got in exchange for all the *good* aspects of drinking are of a deeper void-filling value that I could chase for all eternity in a bottle of red wine or a bag and never find. Life is going to be a slog regardless. Before, I was just numbing myself through the good bits and the bad. I'm saying this next bit cautiously as I might open myself up to ridicule, but the high I get these days from simply standing and watching the sun go down is almost transcendental. I'm not going to compare it to cocaine because obviously one of those things is cocaine. But going out for a walk with the dog in the late evening and knowing that my life is not on fire is one of the simple treasures of this new era that has yet to tarnish. Feeling connected to myself and those around me, knowing that I am loved and capable of unselfishly loving others, not harming myself or consciously causing pain to anybody else – that's the magic stuff that connects me now.

I've also been fortunate enough to witness some profound acts of kindness, courage and love among friends in recovery that make it very easy to connect to something greater than myself. I'm about to use the cliché of all clichés, so please bear with me ... but ... *you never know what sort of day someone is having.* There have been times in the last two and a half years when I have been overwhelmed by life, floored by what can sometimes feel like the terminal prison sentence that is trying to stay sober, when suddenly another alcoholic will pat me lightly on the shoulder, look me in the eye and say, 'Mark, you're doing great!' Seemingly tiny gestures like this have probably saved my life on a couple of occasions, when I have been closer to a drink than I would care to admit. Connection is the opposition of addiction, after all. Now, I don't care for the endless debatable interpret-ations of the word God or what it represents, but for me, connecting to something larger than myself (aka God) is everything. Great OutDoors,

Groups Of Drunks, Good Orderly Direction, Grow Or Die ... whatever. It can be whatever it wants, as long as it's something bigger than me. It doesn't even need to be theological. God just rolls off the tongue and as a concept is familiar to most of us.

MYTH:

I will never be able to enjoy going to concerts again or experience the true elation of music.

REALITY:

When I first gave up alcohol, I felt like I was relearning everything all over again and I remember feeling worried that my sobriety would be too obvious if I ventured out and about, as if I AM AN ALCOHOLIC was written in block capitals across my forehead.

I thought people would be gawking at me when I walked into restaurants, thinking to themselves, 'Oh wow, look at this extraordinary idiot who just came in. He can't drink any more, can't you tell by his disposition? Perhaps that's why he looks so nervous! We should probably all swivel around in our *chairs now and stare at him until he finds his seat. I hope he does something weird!'* I became quite self-conscious – conflating sobriety with weakness – and assumed my recovery was something that I should be ashamed of. I didn't go to the theatre, events or gigs, worried that a member of security might approach me from the side and say, *'Excuse me, sir, but myself and my colleague in the hi-vis over there noticed that you look very uncomfortable in your own skin. Is this because you're sober? Would you mind just stepping this way, please, sir? There's no need for a scene, sir ... Look, you can either come with us quietly or–'* On bad days, it felt like I was 14 years old again, on the banks of the River Dodder, just outside the group, knowing that there was a party happening but not knowing how to get in. When my addiction gets loud, my brain tells me that a good life is *just* out of arm's reach and all it would take to summon a world of happiness would be to walk into the nearest bar, sink eight or ten pints of Guinness, text a dealer, smoke 40 Marlboro Lights, go back to my apartment, buy three bottles of red, get another bag and then sit at my computer all night posting weird Instagram stories and listening to MF DOOM. Alcoholism is a disease of grave deception and amnesia as much as it is of drinking.

In reality, that is total nonsense. Nobody is thinking about me when I go to these places. My experience of music, live or otherwise, in sobriety is as powerful as it's always been. I went to Garth Brooks in September 2022 with *the most outrageous man*, who laughed down the phone at me, and I'm pretty sure that we both had a spiritual experience. I wish I was joking. It was a cultural, religious, emotional steamroller and a monumental surge of something in the soul. I guarantee you even the most staunch critics of country music – or country people – would have been blown away. To this day, Garth Brooks is one of the greatest performers I've ever seen live, and I have been fortunate enough to see quite a few of the best. The concert came at a time when I hadn't really been out that much. If I went further than Dún Laoghaire I'd break out in hives. The night of Garth, I met my friend in town, his car boot was full of Stetsons and he told me that I was going to wear one. I didn't even have a chance to think (which is always a good thing). We went for sushi and walked through the city, looking ridiculous in our hats and loving every minute of it. To feel part of life, separated from my ego and simply sharing the same experience as other people, without sedation, was unreal.

MYTH:

I will not be able to enjoy social occasions, like weddings.

REALITY:

When I was drinking I was under the impression that weddings were a total waste of time: obscenely overpriced, hideously unsentimental and needlessly competitive displays of opulence, forced down our throats by boastful people in their thirties, solely intent on laying down the gauntlet among their own friends before embarking on a lifetime of keeping up with the Joneses. Today, after two and a half years of sobriety, an enormous amount of self-exploration and a healthy dose of challenging my own prejudices, I can honestly say that I still feel the exact same.

The reality is that weddings are probably boring for most people, apart than a select few, whether or not drink is involved. I am not unique in not wanting to be there. It's not my day and that's the whole point. Sometimes it's important to just shut up, nod along and listen to the bride's father listing off her career achievements like a poorly delivered eulogy, or to dance awkwardly during the basic ritual of waving the napkins over your head when the couple come stomping into the room. It doesn't really matter how much short-term pleasure I get out of the day. It's not always all about me.

During the first six months of my sobriety, I had to decline several invitations to weddings that were important to me. Everything was still a little too raw and uncertain and I just had to put my recovery first. I'm sorry now to have missed them. I was terrified that if I went it would result in one of two outcomes. Either (a) I would drink, probably cause a scene and end up punching or scoring the priest. Regardless, it would result in making the entire day about me. Or (b) I would not drink but I would be so obviously miserable and unable to loosen up that I would inevitably make the day about me, too. These days, I share the same anticipation and nervousness as most people when one of my good friends is getting married – hoping that it won't be a dreaded foreign one. (The wedding, that is, not the person they're marrying: I haven't descended into hate speech and decided to roll out a few slurs just as we approach the finishing line.) But the beauty is that I can now say yes to things and know that I will show up, be on time and help out if need be. The freedom from the mortification of perpetually making every single social gathering surreptitiously about me is an extraordinary gift of recovery.

MYTH:

I won't be the same, funny person any more.

REALITY:

Wasn't that the whole idea? Either way, notwithstanding writing a book documenting my alcoholism, fundamental issues of self-worth and matters of the existential variety, I like to think that I am a light enough guy.

A friend of mine, the artist Joshua Gordon, once said in an interview, 'I want to try everything and I don't believe that anyone should limit themselves to one medium.' That's it, really.

Everything is always evolving and I never want to stand still artistically. If humour needed to be sacrificed in the short term so that I could become healthier between the ears, then so be it.

I still worry too much over what everybody thinks about me. 'Everybody' in itself is a very dangerous word. Who is everybody, anyway? And why do I seem to care about them? My brain can convince me of dangerous things when I start thinking too much about 'everybody'.

And I'm fairly sure I read somewhere before – you can't please 'everybody'.

MYTH:

I will never be able to enjoy Christmas.

REALITY:

If every time I went drinking felt like a miniature Christmas, well, you can only imagine how I felt at actual Christmas.

Usually it would start around late October. I'd almost be encouraging people to get their trees up in time for Halloween. It was the season of 'cosy pints' and 'catch-up pints' and it was my

favourite time of the year. Christmas repre-
sented a unique lawlessness, an *anything goes*
period on the drinking calendar, and it was
like crack cocaine for people like me – people
who enjoyed the craic. And the cocaine. It was
a month-long behemoth affair and a marathon
of boozing. Usually, by the time New Year's Eve
rolled around, I would already be bedbound, in
a state of complete shambles. Emotionally, spiritually and financially broken. I'd lie in bed until
the New Year with a frenzied head, wondering
how it had all come and gone without having
anything to show for it. I would be ashamed of
myself for spending the few festive weeks with
all the wrong people and not making one bit of
effort to be around the ones I truly love.

As a boy I adored Christmas. Everything
about it. The anticipation. The sense of magic.
The togetherness. Thanks to my recovery I've
rediscovered the warm feelings I used to have
around the festive season. Within reason, of
course. My family still drive me demented and
there will always be a few arguments thrown
into the mix. It's a highly sensitive time, particularly when you're trying to show your relations
just how different and evolved you are since the

last time they saw you, only to regress into your 14-year-old self upon the first lick of a Brussels sprout or problematic comment from your uncle.

Originally, I wanted to call this chapter 'Help Your *Self Love*'; I thought that it might be an appropriate parting message for the book, an inspirational closing chapter with a nice witty bit of wordplay. Something that perfectly conveys the importance of self-intervention and care when one finds oneself in a pickle or a bind, be it emotional, mental or spiritual. Then I realised that the central point of this whole journey so far, the one lesson, moral, message or learning that leaps out at me from every single low point of my life, is the complete opposite of that. The first and only step towards peace or inner contentment is when I forfeit control, move away from *self* and let the love of the world in. 'Fuck Yourself, Love Others' might have been a better title. But we know how I feel about self-help books with curse words in their title, don't we? Of paramount importance, however, is to remember that the only role I have had in my recovery has been giving up. All it took was one moment of true surrender and the rest was down to the support of others. 'Help' is a very little word with the most beautiful and contagious consequences. I just had to surrender and let their love in.

Aside from that first defeat and loosely following some basic instructions thereafter, my involvement in my recovery overall has been minimal. I have depended entirely on the help of other people when learning how to love myself, how to stay sober, how to grow, how to recover; and how to live. If it weren't for the unconditional wisdom, kindness, friendship, understanding and gentle compassion of every other alcoholic I have been fortunate enough to cross paths with over the last couple of years, I can't imagine what devastating juncture my life would be at today. Who would have thought that talking to drunks would make me not want to drink?

My average morning when drinking was spent cursing myself in the shower. Before I even stepped out onto the street to go to work, I would have had a war of words with myself, blaming my brain for breaking yet another promise and for all of the things I had said or done the night before. Sustenance came in the form of several quickly smoked cigarettes, and potentially a yoghurt, before availing of the free tea or coffee at work.

At weekends, I would lie in bed like a large, greasy baby, sliding around the mattress because I'd have Deliveroo'd a bucket of KFC chicken straight from Earls Court right into the back of my gullet. I'd like to say that the stains on my sheets were remnants of fake tan, worn into the bed linen from intense sex with fleeting love interests, but in reality most of them were from spilled cartons of gravy or spicy mayonnaise from the KFC Tower Burger Zinger Meal. I was absolutely grotesque.

Mornings were a period of recuperation and regret. There was always a stark juxtaposition between the boisterous man I had been the night before versus the meek, trembling boy afraid to get out of bed the following day.

My mornings now are very different. When I am 'on beam' – aka working a good programme of recovery – I begin my day with a gratitude list followed by some meditation. Ten things I am grateful for followed by ten minutes of breath-work/prayer. It helps ground me and prevents my mind boarding the instinctive train of self-obsession. Then I get up and have a cup of coffee. Check my email, text Doireann, text a few alcoholics, read the news, take the dog out for a wee and then get back to the desk. It's all very *quiet*. There is an enormous amount of pleasure to be derived from a noiseless start to the day – internally and externally – and to be comfortable with myself in silence is a gift that is of incalculable worth.

I like getting up early. I always did as a child. I'm not a great man for lying in bed for hours on end. (Unless there's a bucket of fried chicken on the go.) The morning is my favourite part of the day. I look forward to that first coffee with the anticipation that vaguely resembles my former desire for a beer. I'm still an addict to my core but at least for now I am a healthy one. Generally speaking.

One for the road

Each of these practices, and the willingness to persist with them, stems directly from my fear of returning to where I was in the past. And that could happen tomorrow. All I've got are the next 24 hours. Every minute of meditation, self-exploration and myth debunking goes right out the window the moment I pick up that first drink. Whether I return to where I was or descend even further into an oblivion of the terminal variety will remain unclear. But it is a risk that today I believe is not worth taking. Just for today, I know that I am worth more.

But you don't need to know that. You just need to know that you are worth more than the pain you might be experiencing. It might not be booze. Maybe that's not your thing. It could be anything. Sex, relationships, social media, food, gambling, jealousy, anxiety, weight, flying, gossip, Xanax, memory, hypochondria, memory, anger, rage, heroin, memory. It might be a bit of everything. Once I thoroughly re-examined the way I looked at my life and my mental health, and stopped waiting for a diagnosis or an intervention before doing anything about the way I felt, everything began to get incrementally better. Everybody needs a therapist, I think. I'm sure that it's clear to you from reading this book that I'm not exactly a beacon of wellbeing, either. I've still got flaws coming out of my ears. My attitude and outlook on life fluctuate all the time. But I think that's okay and probably an important factor of this book, too. All of this stuff is non-linear and anything less than 'overcoming' or 'completion' does not constitute failure. It's okay to exist in the grey! One setback is not the end of the world. I am better today than I was five years ago, and that's good enough. No matter what happens, *I am good enough*. And so are you, by the way. You are enough. You are more than enough today and you will be more than enough tomorrow. Even if you cannot fully shake the demons. That's okay too.

We don't need to jog on the perennial treadmill of self-betterment until the day we die.

People often commend me for being in recovery. They use the words 'brave' and 'courageous'. What they don't realise is that this was the *easier option*. It was easier to give up than to go on. Going into recovery was stepping in out of the rain. Is there courage in defeat? I don't know. The wellness world would have you believe that it's possible to be cured of everything. My happiness comes from knowing and accepting I will never be cured of anything! This book won't get you well, but if it pushes you to take some steps to get yourself well, fantastic. I am not a life coach and I do not have any of the answers. That's life. Nobody has the answers, and prophets are dangerous. I spent too much of my life putting people on pedestals and they almost always turned out to disappoint me.

The original intention, or myth, of this book was to inspire people who found themselves in a similar position to mine. Lost individuals in their twenties and thirties who couldn't get their shit together. I thought that maybe I had accrued enough wisdom in my short stint of sobriety that it might be worth imparting to others ... Nonsense. After writing this, I've learned that the reality of this book is that it's not about my insights or perspective. It's not about my words or the way I view the world. I've tried to be funny for most of it and at times a bit poetic – which probably came across as clumsy and overly sentimental. It's about zooming out and learning from what I didn't do. I'm just an example of a person who was circling the drain internally and hurtling towards a dark place for a very long time, but thanks to breaking the cycle and doing things differently just once – asking for help – my entire life has changed. One day at a time.

There is no quick fix. It took me a long time to get sick, so it will take me a long time to get better. I'm still a work in progress – a *worth in progress* if you will. And that's it. That's all I have to say for now. So, please, send the text, pick up the phone, write the email. Get rigorously honest with yourself about how you really are. Be less polite when asking friends how they are. If something is off, ask for help. If someone is off, ask them if they need help. It's out there in abundance and you are definitely not alone. You're just not that special. *Nobody* is. And no one else is ever thinking about you as much as you are thinking about you. That's a fact. People aren't mind readers either, so sometimes you'll have to spell it out if you're struggling. You've got to want the change for you, because at the end of the day, you're the one who has to sleep inside your head at night. I wish you well.

Oh, and if all else fails, try to remember:

Focus on what's within. Surround yourself with good people. Try to be more forgiving of yourself. Allow yourself to experience pain. You deserve joy and happiness. Get out of your own way and embrace the imperfections. Switch the phone off every now and then. Reconnect with nature. Remember it's okay to feel overwhelmed by life. By technology. By love. By everything. Suffering isn't endless. You are not alone.

ACKNOWLEDGEMENTS

Thank you to Dave H for picking up the phone and telling me everything would be okay as long as I didn't take a drink that night. You were right. Every person that gets the opportunity to meet you is immediately more wise as a result, of that I am sure. Thank you for everything that you do. It is a privilege to know you.

Rudi, I would not be sober today if it wasn't for you. You picked up the pieces and put them back together more times than I care to admit. Your presence in my life has kept the proverbial lights on even at the darkest of times. I owe you more than words. Thank you.

Paul C – it's an honour to walk this path with you. You are a dear friend and we have learned so much together. Thank you for your friendship.

Theo, the support and encouragement you showed me whilst writing this book is something that I feel deeply unworthy of. You are an innately kind soul and I am grateful to have you as a friend. We're probably lucky we didn't meet in our former lives but I am glad to have you as part of this one. Thank you.

Stuart, you are the best friend I have ever had. Thank you for everything, mate. And that's what you get, Mrs Deady. Let's do the idea.

Doireann, thank you for pushing me to write this book and standing patiently over my shoulder as I did so, even when it got in the way of holidays, weekends away and precious time together. Thank you for helping me get out of my head and forcing me to grow. I love you. You are the most beautiful and gifted person that I have ever known. Although this book mostly covers the past, my future is now yours. Here's to the next adventure.

Mum, rest assured, things are so much better now! A day doesn't go by where I don't feel enormously lucky to have you as a mother. And that's before we even address your secondary roles of friend, therapist, travel companion and Christmas decoration shopping partner. You are an astonishing individual and I still learn from you. I love you. Thank you for everything you do for me.

Dad, you have come to my rescue too many times to mention, thank you. And in the end, you were right about Brighton too! I didn't lick my love for words or my sense of humour off the stones in the street. A walk on Dún Laoghaire pier will always suffice in exchange for a quiet pint in the winter.

Caroline, Freddie, Michelle – fair play to ye.

Lorraine, we both know there's a whole other

book ready to print with the secrets you have up your sleeve, so I won't say too much here! Thank you for treating me with love and kindness throughout some of my most difficult days. You were the life raft that kept me afloat more times than I can even remember.

Thank you to Laura for the support and friendship. I will miss us getting hammered together but wouldn't exchange what we have now for the world. You are a legend.

Ben, our paths don't cross as often as I would like anymore, but those conversations at the beginning of this process were instrumental in giving me the confidence to continue writing. Thank you, mate. The boys down the allegiance would be proud. 'Renny thing left'.

Martin Kelly: 14 years out of secondary school and I still heard your voice criticising me throughout this book when the writing became too flowery. You were the greatest teacher I ever had and cemented my love for English at a time when I wanted to drop out of school entirely. Thank you.

To my friends in and around Dún Laoghaire: Thank you for loving me when I could not love myself. It's a pleasure to learn from your experience. You give me strength and hope. One day at a time. Thank you.

Thanks to Teresa for taking a chance on this book and helping craft it into something readable. The whole process of working with you has been a pleasure. Your gentle encouragement helped alleviate the near constant sense of imposter syndrome, particularly when doubt would get in the way of writing. Isabelle, thank you for sprinkling your magic and helping finesse this story in ways that I would never have even thought of. You have been an incredibly valuable addition to the process - even when replying with a mere '?' to passages in the book that were supposed to be funny.

Finally, to John. I now understand why I always felt a special bond with you. May I continue to be humbled by and learn from the fortitude you showed in your final days. Rest in peace.

God grant me the serenity to accept the things I cannot change, the courage to change the things I can and the wisdom to know the difference.